Current Topics in Microbiology 156 and Immunology

The Role of Viruses and the Immune System in Diabetes Mellitus

Experimental Models

Edited by T. Dyrberg

With 15 Figures

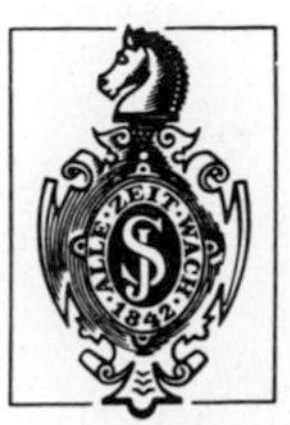

Springer-Verlag
Berlin Heidelberg NewYork
London Paris Tokyo HongKong

THOMAS DYRBERG, M.D.

Hagedorn Research Laboratory,
Niels Steensens Vej 6,
2820 Gentofte, Denmark

ISBN 3-540-51918-1 Springer-Verlag Berlin Heidelberg New York
ISBN 0-387-51918-1 Springer-Verlag New York Berlin Heidelberg

Library of Congress Catalog Card Number 15-12910
Printed in Germany

Phototypesetting: Thomson Press (India) Ltd, New Delhi
Offsetprinting: Saladruck, Berlin; Bookbinding: B. Helm Berlin
2123/3020-543210 – Printed on acid-free paper.

Foreword

Research in diabetes has accelerated in two areas, both of which are being reviewed in CTMI. The first is the use of a variety of animal models; the second is basic research in human investigation, islet cell antigens, and mapping of genes associated with susceptibility to disease. Dr. Thomas Dyrberg accepted editorial responsibility for this volume, which covers the first area. A second book, to be published later in the year, is edited by Drs. Bækkeskov and Hansen (CTMI 164, see page VI for contents). Although the contributors to both volumes represent the international scientific community, the editors are from the Hagedorn Research Laboratory in Denmark. Work at this institute and the Steno Memorial Hospital has been dedicated to research in diabetes for decades, and the institutions were appointed WHO Collaborating Centres for Research and Training on the Pathogenesis of Diabetes Mellitus in 1983. It is worth noting that while addressing the hypothesis of the role of class II major histocompatibility glycoproteins in autoimmune diabetes (insulin-dependent diabetes, IDDM) a number of investigators established animal models in which class II molecules were expressed under the control of the rat insulin promoter. While generating interesting information on IDDM, the finding of immunologic tolerance in such transgenic mice has attracted the attention of several basic immunologic laboratories for quite different reasons. Thus, we are reminded again of the Pasteur dictum that "chance favors the prepared mind."

Michael B. A. Oldstone, M.D.
La Jolla, California, November 1989

This collection of studies was conceived as part of a two-volume review of the immunology of diabetes. The contents of Volume 164, which forms part 2, are listed below.

Current Topics in Microbiology and Immunology, Volume 164

Human Diabetes

(Edited by S. Bækkeskov and B. Hansen)

Preface

Insulin-dependent (type 1) diabetes mellitus (IDDM) is a chronic disease caused by specific destruction of the pancreatic β cells. Replacement therapy with insulin nearly normalizes glucose metabolism; however, IDDM is still associated with excessive mortality due to severe secondary complications. An important aspect of diabetes research is to clarify the etiology and pathogenesis of IDDM. This knowledge may enable us to identify individuals who are beginning to develop diabetes and to intervene in the pathogenic processes, thereby preventing clinical onset of disease. Although the exact mechanisms responsible for β cell destruction have not yet been determined, it is known that:

—Autoimmunity is of major significance in the pathogenesis, but the initial events leading to the break in self-tolerance to β cell autoantigens remain obscure.

—Susceptibility to IDDM is closely associated with certain MHC class II genes, but other genes may also play a role.

—Environmental factors can cause IDDM and are probably important in inducing the initial lesions.

Animal research has had a place in the study of diabetes since Minkowski reported on the pivotal role of the pancreas in the development of diabetes 100 years ago. The three animal models which have been of particular importance for the study of IDDM are reviewed in this volume—low-dose streptozotocin diabetes in mice, the BB rat, and the NOD mouse. The diabetic syndrome of the latter two shares many similarities with IDDM in humans; most prominently they develop diabetes subsequent to autoimmune destruction of their β cells. Studies on the pathogenic mechanisms in these animals may help to uncover mechanisms which are difficult to study in humans such as tolerance and prediabetes pathogenesis.

Although diabetes research has focused on autoimmune phenomena, the association between IDDM and virus needs to be explored further. Viruses have been implicated by various indirect observations, but direct evidence that virus can cause IDDM is limited. Infection with Coxsackie B virus has precipitated an acute onset of IDDM in a few cases. Individuals with congenital rubella infection are particularly prone to develop IDDM, but it remains to be established whether rubella virus is the etiologic agent. Viruses can, however, cause autoimmune disease by multiple mechanisms, either directly, by interacting with the target cells or indirectly, by interfering with the function of the immune system.

Recent developments in molecular genetics have illuminated the role of major histocompatibility complex molecules in IDDM and the genetics of IDDM in the BB rat. These subjects are also reviewed in this volume.

Taken together, it is obvious from the contributions in this book that major advances have been made in understanding the pathogenesis of IDDM, but that a host of questions are still unanswered. In the long run, it will be necessary to improve and enhance the interdisciplinary approach for not until then will it be possible to design effective preventive IDDM therapy.

January 1990 T. Dyrberg

List of Contents

List of Contributors

(Their addresses can be found at the beginning of their respective chapters)

ACHA-ORBEA, H.
ALLISON, J.
CAMPBELL, I. L.
CHATTERJEE, N. K.
CONTREAS, G.
GERLING, I.
HANAFUSA, T.
HARRISON, L. C.
JØRGENSEN, J.
KASTERN, W.
KRYSPIN-SØRENSEN, I.
LANG, F.
LEITHER, E. H.
MADSEN, O. D.
MCDEVITT, H. O.
MILLER, J. A. F. P.
RAYFIELD, E. J.
SCOTT, J.
TARUI, S.
WILSON, G. L.

The Spontaneously Diabetic BB Rat: Sites of the Defects Leading to Autoimmunity and Diabetes Mellitus. A Review

J. Scott

1 Introduction

The spontaneously diabetic BB rat, discovered serendipitously in 1974 in a commercial breeding facility (BioBreeding Laboratories, Ottawa, Ontario), is an animal model that displays clinical and pathologic features closely resembling Type 1 (insulin-dependent, juvenile-onset) diabetes mellitus in humans. In both diseases, an immune pathogenesis appears to contribute to the destruction of the pancreatic beta cells. Since first described by Nakhooda and coworkers (Nakhooda et al. 1977), the BB rat diabetic syndrome has been extensively characterized. The syndrome is manifest by an abrupt onset of severe hyperglycemia secondary to insulinopenia, with a lymphocytic and monocytic infiltration of the pancreatic islets (insulitis) before and during the acute phase of hyperglycemia (Like et al. 1982a; Marliss et al. 1982; Like and Rossini 1984; Yale and Marliss 1984). Genetically susceptible male and female rats develop hyperglycemia with equal frequency and severity, with the time of onset varying from approximately 60 to 120 days of age. Peak onset of diabetes occurs around the age of sexual maturation (80–100 days); the frequency of diabetes in untreated BB rats less than 60 days of age is 0.5% (Like and Rossini 1984). Characteristically, the animals are nonobese, and diabetic animals require daily insulin injections to prevent ketoacidosis and death. As in humans, the diabetic syndrome has been shown to be associated with genes in the major histocompatibility complex (MHC) (Colle et al. 1981; Jackson et al. 1984). No known pathogens have been implicated; the syndrome occurs with equal frequency and severity in animals raised in a pathogen-free environment (Rossini et al. 1979).

As in human Type 1 diabetes, the syndrome in the BB rat develops against a background of heightened autoreactivity, with multiple autoantibodies being detectable during the prediabetic period. These include antibodies of the immunoglobulin G (IgG) class which bind to the islet cell surface, to thyroglobulin, to insulin, and to both skeletal and smooth muscle (Dyrberg et al. 1982; Like et al. 1982a; Elder et al. 1982; Dean et al. 1987). Lymphocyte

Department of Pediatrics, The University of Virginia School of Medicine, Charlottesville, VA 22908, USA

Current Topics in Microbiology and Immunology, Vol. 156

antibodies and gastric parietal cell antibodies are also present (DYRBERG et al. 1982; ELDER et al. 1982). The precise relationship of these autoantibodies to the development of diabetes, however, is uncertain.

In addition to its diabetic syndrome, the BB rat is characterized by a profound T lymphocytopenia, with a marked decrease in both helper/inducer T cells (T_h/T_i) and cytotoxic/suppressor T cells (T_c/T_s) (JACKSON et al. 1981; BELLGRAU et al. 1982; POUSSIER et al. 1982; ELDER and MACLAREN 1983). Although T_c/T_s cells are normally identified by the presence of the 0X8 surface antigen (BRIDEAU et al. 1980), monoclonal antibodies to OX8 also bind to natural killer (NK) cells (CANTRELL et al. 1982). There is an apparent total lack of T_c/T_s cells in the peripheral blood of diabetes-prone BB rats (WODA et al. 1986), with virtually all of the $OX8^+$ cells in diabetes-prone BB rats identified as NK cells by their coexpression of the marker for asialo-GM1 (WODA and BIRON 1986).

As is typical of autoimmunity in other animals, BB rat lymphocytes show depressed responsiveness to alloantigen in the mixed lymphocyte reaction (MLR) (BELLGRAU et al. 1982; ELDER and MACLAREN 1983; SCOTT et al. 1984). Studies of concanavalin A (ConA) responses in BB rats have produced conflicting data (BELLGRAU et al. 1982; JACKSON et al. 1983; YALE and MARLISS 1984; VAREY et al. 1987). The findings by ROSSINI et al. (1979) that responses to ConA were low in rats with insulitis but normal in rats without insulitis may at least partially explain the discrepancies. PRUD'HOMME et al. (1984) attributed this defect to suppressor macrophages. It was originally believed that such T-cell dysfunction might be important for the expression of diabetes in the BB rat. However, we have recently demonstrated (SCOTT et al. 1986a, 1987a, 1989) that neonatal thymectomy in BB rats followed by transplantation of thymuses from MHC-compatible (Wistar-Furth) newborn rats restores in vitro lymphocyte function (on a per T-cell basis) to near normal in the absence of any major effects on total lymphocyte numbers or T-cell subset distributions. Diabetes occurred, however, in animals with normal in vitro responses to alloantigen. Such studies suggested that, at least in part, the in vitro lymphocyte hyporesponsiveness characteristic of BB rats results from a defect in T-cell maturation in the thymus. The studies demonstrated, therefore, that the expression of diabetes in the BB rat is not dependent upon decreased lymphocyte responsiveness.

The precise phenotypic identification of the effector cells that mediate final destruction of the pancreatic beta cells has not been accomplished. However, a cell-mediated autoimmune mechanism of pathogenesis for the condition has been suggested by the presence of the lymphocytic insulitis, the findings that neonatal thymectomy or immunosuppression with antilymphocytic serum effectively prevents and/or ameliorates the disease (LIKE et al. 1979, 1982c) and the demonstration of a sine qua non of autoimmunity, i.e., passive transfer of the disorder from the affected animal to a susceptible recipient by inoculation with ConA-activated spleen cells (KOEVARY et al. 1983, 1985; LIKE et al. 1985). Efforts to transfer the disease with serum have failed (NAJI et al. 1981a).

Evidence that the diabetic syndrome in BB rats is T cell-mediated stems from a number of observations, such as prevention of the disease by neonatal thymectomy (LIKE et al. 1982b) or by transfusions from a diabetes-resistant subline of BB rats of peripheral T lymphocytes enriched for T helper/inducer cells (MORDES et al. 1987). One likely mechanism for prevention of diabetes by normal T_h/T_i cells would be the restoration of a suppressor T-cell circuit. Diabetes can also be prevented by administration of T-cell immunosuppressants such as cyclosporin-A (LIKE et al. 1982c), or by in vivo administration of a monoclonal antibody against the OX19 (T-cell) surface antigen (LIKE et al. 1986). If T cells, therefore, play a role in the pathogenesis of the diabetic syndrome, it then becomes important to ask how these defects in the T-cell compartment originate, and whether they result from an abnormal lymphoid stem cell or from an abnormal differentiative environment.

2 Bone Marrow Chimera Studies

In studies by NAJI and coworkers (NAJI et al. 1981a, 1981b, 1982, 1983), neonatal inoculation of diabetes-prone BB rats with bone marrow from a normal MHC-compatible strain of rat significantly reduced the incidence of diabetes. Using neonatal rats of an outbred colony of BB rats, they showed that in neonatal rats injected with normal Wistar-Furth (WF) bone marrow cells, only 8% subsequently became diabetic, while 41% of noninjected BB rat controls developed the disease. Furthermore, the increased ability of such bone marrow-inoculated rats to subsequently mount alloantigen-specific MLRs was shown to be due to donor-derived T cells. The authors interpreted their results as indicating that diabetes in the BB rat is at leastly partly due to a defect in a lymphoid stem cell precursor. However, it is well established that normal bone marrow contains a population of mature T cells similar to the mature T lymphocyte pool found in peripheral blood; these bone marrow T cells most probably enter the bone marrow parenchyma as part of the normal recirculating lymphocyte pool (HÄAS et al. 1969; FAUCI 1975; ABDOU et al. 1976). The studies by NAJI and coworkers, therefore, did not specifically address the question of which lymphoid cell population was directly responsible for the prevention of diabetes and the restoration of lymphocyte responsiveness in the inoculated recipients. Prevention of disease may have been due to cotransfer of mature T cells in the inoculum, providing suppressor T cells necessary for the control of autoimmune response.

A requirement for mature T cells would suggest a defect in the T-cell differentiative environment (i.e., post stem cell) in BB rats. Conversely, if the defect(s) in the BB rat leading to diabetes resides in the lymphoid stem cell precursors, transferring only stem cells (depleted of mature T cells) from normal MHC-compatible animals into diabetes-prone animals should prevent the onset of diabetes and/or correct the T-cell abnormalities. Our laboratory constructed a series of bone marrow chimeras, using various combinations of normal or BB rat recipients and donors, in an attempt to address this question. Our studies involved the construction of both neonatal (Scott et al. 1986b) and adult (Scott et al. 1987b) chimeras.

2.1 Neonatal Bone Marrow Chimera Studies

Within 36 h after birth, diabetes-prone BB rats were inoculated i.p. with bone marrow from MHC-compatible WF rats (Scott et al. 1986b). For one half of the recipients, the bone marrow inoculum was depleted of mature T cells by treatment with rabbit antirat thymocyte antiserum plus guinea pig complement. At time of killing, cytofluorographic analyses of spleen cells were performed on a fluorescence-activated cell sorter by incubation with murine-derived monoclonal antibodies to surface antigens W3/13 (T cells and neutrophils), OX19 (T cells), W3/25 (T_h/T_i cells and macrophages), and OX8 (T_c/T_s and NK cells), followed by incubation with a fluorescein isothiocyanate-conjugated $F(ab')_2$ fragment of goat antimouse IgG. Lymphocyte function was assessed by 5-day mixed lymphocyte reactions (MLRs) using allogeneic (Fisher) rat spleen cells as stimulators, and 3-day ConA stimulation assays.

Table 1 summarizes the results of our neonatal bone marrow chimera studies. As in the earlier study by Naji and coworkers described above, those animals receiving untreated (whole) WF bone marrow showed a decreased incidence of diabetes, with only 23% of the inoculated BB neonates becoming diabetic by 140 days of age ($P < 0.005$, compared with the 68% incidence observed in BB controls). The inoculated animals also showed a restoration of lymphocyte in vitro responsiveness ($P < 0.05$ and $P < 0.01$, compared with BB controls, for MLR and ConA responses, respectively). The reduced incidence of diabetes in these animals, however, appeared to be unrelated to the extent of lymphopenia.

Table 1. Diabetes incidence, lymphopenia, and lymphocyte in vitro responsiveness in BB rats injected neonatally with WF bone marrow

BB rat group	Diabetes incidence (%)	Lymphocytes/μl $\times 10^{-3}$	MLR response $\times 10^{-3}$ (cpm)[a]	ConA response $\times 10^{-3}$ (cpm)[a]
BB controls	68	3.55 ± 0.54(12)	2.86 ± 0.40(5)	22.08 ± 2.44(15)
Recipients of untreated WF bone marrow	23*	4.94 ± 0.79**(16)	15.61 ± 4.88***(6)	50.93 ± 8.13****(8)
Recipients of T cell-depleted WF bone marrow	75[†]	3.05 ± 0.54(11)	ND	ND

Animals are as described in the text. Lymphocyte data are expressed as means ± SEM. Analyses were conducted at time of death, ~ 150 days of age or within 2–3 weeks after onset of diabetes. Numbers in parentheses indicate the number of rats examined. *$P < 0.005$ compared with BB controls; **$P < 0.02$ compared with BB controls, by analysis of variance; ***$P < 0.05$ compared with BB controls, by t test; ****$P < 0.01$ compared with BB controls, by t test. [†]NS compared with BB controls. [a]Spleen cells were plated in the presence of either ConA or allogeneic spleen cells, in medium containing 5% horse serum; responsiveness was assessed by the subsequent incorporation of ^{3}H-thymidine

Although these animals showed a small improvement in lymphocyte counts, regardless of whether or not they became diabetic, they were still significantly leukopenic and lymphopenic compared with WF controls. In contrast, 75% of the BB neonates inoculated with T cell-depleted bone marrow became diabetic, an incidence not significantly different from that in BB controls ($P > 0.10$). Inoculation of T cell-depleted bone marrow did not significantly affect T-cell subset distributions (data not shown). The inability of T cell-depleted bone marrow to prevent diabetes in these studies suggests the presence of a defect in the T-cell differentiative environment in BB rats, i.e., either a thymic or postthymic defect.

2.2 Bone Marrow Irradiation Chimera Studies

In a further attempt to determine the site of the defect(s) leading to diabetes and/or lymphopenia in the BB rat, our laboratory carried out bone marrow chimera studies in adult (> 37 days of age) rats (Scott et al. 1987b). Each recipient was given 800 rad whole-body irradiation; within 6 h of irradiation, recipients were injected i.c. with 5×10^7 T cell-depleted bone marrow cells. A total of 52 diabetes-prone BB rats, 40–109 days of age, were inoculated with WF bone marrow (WF → BB chimeras); 23 WF rats were inoculated with bone marrow from overtly diabetic BB donors (BB → WF chimeras); 21 adolescent diabetes-prone BB rats were inoculated with bone marrow from overtly diabetic BB donors, as irradiation controls (BB → BB "chimeras"); and 7 adolescent WF rats were inoculated with WF bone marrow (WF → WF "chimeras"). All animals were observed for over 140 days post inoculation, or until diabetes onset. A monoclonal antibody to the RT-7.2 T-cell differentiation alloantigen, generously donated by Dr. D.L. Greiner (University of Connecticut Health Center,

Table 2. Diabetes incidence, lymphopenia, and lymphocyte in vitro responsiveness in BB rat bone marrow irradiation chimeras

Rat group	Diabetes incidence (%)	Lymphocytes/μl $\times 10^{-3}$	MLR (% of values for WF controls)[a]
WF → WF chimeras	0	7.65 ± 0.74(5)	ND
BB → WF chimeras	0	7.97 ± 0.51(5)	−93 ± 4(6)
WF → BB chimeras	0*	9.10 ± 0.90(18)	−93 ± 19(10)
BB → BB chimeras	24**	3.22 ± 0.30***(19)	−5 ± 5***(16)
BB litter-matched controls	38	3.45 ± 0.36(21)	−2 ± 1(13)

Animals are as described in the text. Lymphocyte counts are expressed as means ± SEM. Number in parentheses indicates the number of rats examined. MLR, mixed lymphocyte reaction; *$P < 0.007$ compared with BB → BB litter-matched irradiation chimeras; **NS compared with litter-matched BB controls; ***$P < 0.0001$ compared with WF controls (data not shown), NS compared with litter-matched BB controls. [a]Spleen cells were plated in the presence of irradiated allogeneic spleen cells, in medium containing 10% fetal calf serum; results are expressed as the cpm of ^{3}H-thymidine incorporated, divided by the cpm incorporated by WF lymphocytes, × 100

Farmington), was used to document the persistence of donor-origin lymphoid cells in the WF → BB chimeras; the RT-7.2 antigen is totally absent on BB rat lymphoid cells (GREINER et al. 1986).

Table 2 summarizes the results of our bone marrow irradiation chimera studies in adult rats. Diabetes occurred in 24% of the BB → BB chimeras, an incidence not significantly different than the 38% incidence in litter-matched controls ($P > 0.05$). If followed by immunologic reconstitution, therefore, irradiation per se does not appear to significantly affect the incidence of diabetes. Lymphopenia and lymphocyte in vitro responsiveness in the BB → BB chimeras were comparable to untreated BB control rats. As might be predicted, none of the WF rats irradiated and injected with T cell-depleted WF bone marrow (WF → WF chimeras) developed either diabetes or lymphopenia.

None of the WF rats irradiated and injected with marrow from overtly diabetic BB rats (BB → WF chimeras) developed diabetes or lymphopenia; their lymphocytes demonstrated normal MLR responsiveness compared with WF controls. The failure to induce diabetes and/or lymphocyte abnormalities in this group indicated that BB bone marrow stem cells can differentiate in an apparently normal fashion in an irradiated normal host.

In all irradiated BB rats that had received T cell-depleted WF bone marrow (WF → BB chimeras), spleen cells were positive for the RT-7.2 differentiation alloantigen, verifying the persistence of donor-origin lymphoid cells and thus documenting the chimeric state. The incidence of diabetes in irradiated BB rats injected with WF bone marrow (WF → BB chimeras) was significantly reduced ($P < 0.001$ compared with untreated control BB rats), with zero incidence of diabetes (0/32) in animals that were less than 44 days of age at time of bone marrow transfer. This latter group had normal lymphocyte counts and MLR responsiveness, compared with WF controls. Surprisingly, however, WF → BB chimeras did not show complete normalization of their T-cell subset distributions (data nor shown); although the proportions of cells in the $0X19^+$, $W3/13^+$, and $W3/25^+$ subsets were significantly increased compared to values in BB controls, these subsets were still significantly decreased compared to WF and WF → WF control rats. The proportion of $0X8^+$ cells was only slightly greater than that of BB → BB chimeras ($P < 0.04$).

Let us compare the WF → BB chimeras with the BB → BB chimeras: only their [donor] bone marrow stem cells differ; their T-cell differentiative environment is identical. Prevention of diabetes in the WF → BB chimeras appears, therefore, to be the result of the correction of a stem-cell defect. Let us now compare, however, the BB → WF chimeras with the BB → BB chimeras: only their T-cell differentiative environments differ; their [donor] bone marrow stem cells are identical. Inoculation with [abnormal] BB stem cells failed to induce diabetes and/or lymphocyte abnormalities in the BB → WF chimeras. Apparently the stem-cell defect evidenced by the WF → BB chimeras is a necessary-but-not-sufficient defect for diabetes expression in an animal with a normal T-cell differentiative environment. Moreover, the failure to completely restore the T-cell subsets in WF → BB chimeras could be interpreted as additional evidence for a defective T-cell differentiative environment in the diabetes-prone BB rat, as was suggested in our neonatal bone marrow chimera studies.

In more recently reported studies, NAKANO and coworkers constructed bone marrow irradiation chimeras using combinations of diabetes-prone and diabetes-resistant BB/Wor rats (NAKANO et al. 1988). The diabetes-prone BB recipients were 28–32 days old at time of irradiation/inoculation; the diabetes-resistant BB recipients were 30–280 days of age, with all but six over 60 days of age. Of the diabetes-prone recipients of diabetes-prone bone marrow 30% became diabetic, results comparable to our studies described above. As might be predicted, none of the diabetes-resistant recipients of diabetes-resistant bone marrow became diabetic. None of the diabetes-prone recipients of diabetes-resistant bone marrow became diabetic. These results are comparable to our studies described above, in which none of the diabetes-prone recipients of WF bone marrow (if less than 44 days of age at time of transfer) became diabetic. In contrast, 25% of the diabetes-resistant recipients of diabetes-prone bone marrow developed the disease. In our studies, normal MHC-compatible WF recipients of diabetic bone marrow did not become diabetic. The studies of NAKANO and coworkers suggest, therefore, that unlike normal WF rats, diabetes-resistant BB/W or rats harbor an effector cell population capable of beta-cell destruction.

Taken together, our bone marrow chimera studies (SCOTT et al. 1986b, 1987b) and those of others suggest that there are two defects in the BB rat associated with the expression of diabetes. One defect occurs at the level of the bone marrow stem cell, and the other resides within the T-cell differentiative environment.

3 Thymus Transplantation Studies

The defect in the T-cell differentiative environment suggested by our bone marrow chimera studies could reside either within the thymus or in the postthymic compartment of T-cell maturation. If the defect resides within the thymus itself, transplantation of normal thymuses from MHC-compatible rats into diabetes-prone BB rats should prevent diabetes and/or lymphopenia. As discussed previously, BB rat lymphocytes show depressed responsiveness to alloantigen in MLRs (BELLGRAU et al. 1982; ELDER and MACLAREN 1983; SCOTT et al. 1984), and responses to ConA are often low (ROSSINI et al. 1979b; BELLGRAU et al. 1982; JACKSON et al. 1983; YALE and MARLISS 1984; PRUD'HOMME et al. 1984; VAREY et al. 1987). If thymus transplantations corrected the lymphocyte hyporesponsiveness characteristic of BB rats, would such restoration be necessarily accompanied by prevention of diabetes, i.e., how important is the T-cell dysfunction for the expression of diabetes in the BB rat?

3.1 Thymus Transplants in Neonatal Recipients

Our laboratory grafted newborn WF thymuses into the vicinity of the thyroid gland of 44 neonatal (<2 days of age) diabetes-prone BB rats (SCOTT et al. 1986a, 1987a, 1989). We reasoned, however, that if the [putative] thymic defect were exerting a dominant effect, recipients of such normal thymuses might still manifest the defect (and become diabetic and/or lymphopenic) due to the presence of their endogenous thymus. Therefore, our thymus graft recipients were thymectomized immediately prior to transplant. The animal groups consisted of 28 "sham"-operated BB neonates as controls, 27 BB neonates that were thymectomized only, and 44 BB littermates that were thymectomized and grafted with neonatal WF thymuses. All animals were followed for over 195 days of age, or until diabetes onset.

Table 3 illustrates the effects of neonatal thymectomy and thymus grafting in diabetes-prone BB rats. As reported earlier by LIKE et al. (1982b), there was a marked reduction in incidence of diabetes in thymectomized-only rats compared with litter-matched shams, even in those animals documented to have received only partial thymectomies (no diabetes occurred in completely thymectomized animals). Thymus grafts, however, had no apparent effect on diabetes incidence: the thymectomized/thymus-grafted BB rats showed a slight, but not statistically significant reduction in incidence compared with shams. Moreover, diabetes occurred in 50% of the thymectomized/thymus-grafted animals documented to have received complete thymectomies. As shown in Table 3, thymus grafting also had no apparent effect on peripheral blood lymphopenia, nor on splenic T-cell

Table 3. Effects of neonatal thymectomy and thymus transplants on diabetes incidence, lymphopenia, and lymphocyte in vitro responsiveness in BB rats

Rat group	Diabetes incidence (%)	Lymphocytes/ $\mu l \times 10^{-3}$	MLR[a] (% of WF values)	ConA response[a] (% of WF values)
Surgical "sham" BBs	43	2.94 ± 0.33 (13)	26 ± 7* (12)	33 ± 6* (8)
Thymectomized/thymus-grafted BBs	30**	2.54 ± 0.14** (43)	$71 + 9$ (32)	ND
Complete thymectomy	50**	2.85 ± 0.27** (8)	79 ± 17*** (6)	74 ± 7***** (6)
Thymectomized-Only BBs	11[†]	2.81 ± 0.32 (25)	5 ± 1* (22)	ND
Complete thymectomy	0[†]	1.46 ± 0.11[‡] (5)	4 ± 1* (4)	30 ± 8* (3)
WF controls	—	10.53 ± 0.58 (36)	100 (26)	100 (8)

Animals are as described in the text. Lymphocyte counts are expressed as means ± SEM; number in parentheses indicates the number of rats examined. MLR, mixed lymphocyte reaction; * $P < 0.0001$ compared with WF controls. ** NS compared with shams, by analysis of variance; *** NS compared with WF controls and $P < 0.003$ compared with shams; **** $P < 0.0001$ compared with shams and $P < 0.0007$ compared with WF controls. [†] $P < 0.01$ compared with shams, by analysis of variance; [‡] $P < 0.0001$ (by two-tailed t test) compared with comparable animals (completely thymectomized) in the thymectomized/thymus-grafted group. [a] T cell-enriched spleen cells were plated in the presence of either ConA or irradiated allogeneic spleen cells, in medium containing 10% fetal calf serum; results are expressed as the cpm of ^{3}H-thymidine incorporated, divided by the cpm incorporated by WF lymphocytes, × 100 subset distributions (data not shown). The grafting of a normal thymus did have, however, a striking effect on lymphocyte in vitro responsiveness. T cell-enriched lymphocytes from completely thymectomized/thymus-grafted or partially thymectomized/thymus-grafted rats demonstrated normal or near normal MLR values, respectively. A dominant role played by the BB thymus in controlling lymphocyte dysfunction is suggested by comparing these two groups of thymus-grafted animals. These studies suggest that, at least in part, the in vitro lymphocyte hyporesponsiveness characteristic of diabetes-prone BB rats may result from a defect in T-cell maturation in the thymus. Of particular interest was the observation that diabetes occurred in lymphopenic animals with normal lymphocyte in vitro responsiveness. Thus, the expression of diabetes in lymphopenic BB rats is not dependent upon abnormal lymphocyte responsiveness.

The findings that thymus graft recipients developed overt diabetes at the same frequency as their nongrafted, nonthymecotmized littermates, and the observation that both groups remain lymphopenic, suggest that the defects responsible for the onset of diabetes and T-cell lymphopenia in the BB rat do not reside in the thymus. The defect in the T-cell differentiative environment suggested by our bone marrow chimera studies, therefore, apparently resides in the postthymic compartment of T-cell maturation.

3.2 Thymus Transplants in Adult Recipients

In studies by Francfort and coworkers (Francfort et al. 1985), thymuses were transplanted into adult diabetes-prone rats from a nondiabetes-prone subline of BB rats. In similar studies, recently reported by Georgiou and coworkers (Georgiou et al. 1988), thymuses were transplanted from fetal DA/BB F_1 rats into adult diabetes-prone BB recipients. As in our neonatal thymus recipient studies described above, the grafting of nondiabetes-prone thymuses into diabetes-prone animals in both of these latter studies did not restore lymphocyte subset distributions to normal. Thus, all three studies argue against the thymus as the site of the defect leading to T-cell lymphopenia in this animal model.

In the studies by Georgiou and coworkers, MLR responses in the thymus graft recipients approached the range of normal rats, despite the lack of restoration of T-cell subsets. Thymectomized/thymus-grafted animals demonstrated lymphocyte in vitro responsiveness that declined with time, i.e., from 7 weeks post transplantation (16 weeks of age) to 16 weeks post transplantation (25 weeks of age). Georgiou and coworkers interpreted this decline in T-cell in vitro function as a consequence of repopulation of the thymus grafts with bone marrow-derived BB rat non-T-cell precursors. In contrast, in our neonatal thymus transplantation studies described above, normal T-cell in vitro function was demonstrated in rats with thymus grafts of long duration, i.e., means of 22 weeks and 37 weeks post transplantation for overtly diabetic rats and for nondiabetic littermates, respectively. There are several important differences in the two studies, however: (1) The age of the graft recipients: Our animals were thymectomized within 36 h of birth and immediately given thymus grafts; the rats in the study by GEORGIOU and coworkers were thymectomized at 7 weeks of age, lethally irradiated and bone marrow reconstituted at 8 weeks of age, and thymus grafted at 9 weeks of age. (2) The source of donor thymus: In our study, normal MHC-compatible (WF) neonatal rats served as thymus donors; in the study by GEORGIOU and coworkers, the donors were fetal DA/BB F_1 hybrids. (3) The source of the graft recipients: Our diabetes-prone graft recipients were derived from the breeding nucleus at the University of Massachusetts; the diabetes-prone recipients in the study by GEORGIOU and coworkers were derived from the breeding nucleus at the University of Philadelphia. It is known that genetic heterogeneity exists between different BB rat subpopulations, affecting incidence, age at onset, untreated survival time of diabetes, lymphopenia, and body weight gain (KLÖTING et al. 1987). (4) The source of lymphoid tissue used for the in vitro functional assay differed in the two studies.

The numbers of grafted animals in the study by FRANCFORT and coworkers and in the study by GEORGIOU and coworkers were too small to evaluate effects of the thymus grafts on diabetes incidence.

4 RT6 T Lymphocyte Differentiation Antigen Studies

Recent reports have suggested that T lymphocytes expressing the differentiation alloantigen RT6 are important regulators of the autoimmune process in the BB rat (ROSSINI et al. 1986; BURSTEIN et al. 1989). RT6 is expressed on the surface of most peripheral T lymphocytes, but is not expressed on thymic lymphocytes or bone marrow cells. During the maturation of T lymphocytes in the lymph nodes of normal rats, the thymic marker Thy-1 is lost and the RT6 marker appears. $RT6^+$ T cells appear late in ontogeny and do not reach maximal levels until rats are 40–50 days of age (THIELE et al. 1987; MOJCIK et al. 1988). Normal rats express RT6 on approximately 60% of their peripheral T cells (ELY et al. 1983). WF rat lymphocytes express the RT6.2 T-cell antigen, lymphocytes from the diabetes-resistant subline of BB/Wor rats express RT6.1, and diabetes-prone BB/Wor rat lymphocytes have been reported to express neither RT6 antigen (GREINER et al. 1986). When a monoclonal antibody directed against RT6 was used to deplete the $RT6^+$ cells from diabetes-resistant BB rats, animals developed insulitis and/or diabetes (GREINER et al. 1987). Induction of diabetes by depletion of $RT6^+$ cells in diabetes-resistant BB rats raises the question of whether a defective gene for RT6 could be the cause of lymphopenia and/or diabetes in diabetes-prone BB rats.

Recent studies in the laboratory of Dr. WILLIAM KASTERN at the University of Florida College of Medicine, Gainesville, took advantage of the close linkage between the RT6 and albino genes on rat chromosome 1 (O'BRIEN 1987) to test the role of the RT6 gene in the inheritance of lymphopenia and diabetes in BB rats (personal communication, W. KASTERN, unpublished results). KASTERN performed outcrosses between a diabetic BB rat and a Long Evans Hooded rat; the segregation of the RT6 gene was studied in 207 F_2 animals. For an F_2 animal to be albino required that both homologues of chromosome 1 come from the diabetes-prone BB grandparent. Although most of the albino F_2 rats should have been homozygous for the BB RT6 gene, KASTERN found no increase in the incidence of diabetes or lymphopenia among albino F_2 rats when compared to their hooded littermates. Only 22.2% of the albino F_2 rats developed lymphopenia, and only 3.7% developed diabetes. KASTERN interprets these results as indicating that the RT6 gene is not linked to diabetes or lymphopenia in the BB rat. To investigate whether the expression of RT6 could be specifically altered in diabetic rats, RT6 expression on peripheral blood lymphocytes was investigated within the entire F_2 generation. No difference was observed in RT6 expression between albinos and their hooded littermates, suggesting that the BB RT6 gene was able to be fully functional and expressed normally on the surface of T cells.

The unpublished results of these studies by KASTERN suggest that neither a defective RT6 gene nor altered expression of the RT6 antigen account for diabetes or lymphopenia in diabetes-prone rats. Further studies will be needed to confirm or refute these findings.

5 Summary

In summary, our bone marrow chimeras studies suggest that there are two defects in the BB rat associated with diabetes and/or lymphopenia, one residing at the level of the bone marrow lymphoid stem cell and the other within the T-cell differentiative environment, apparently postthymic. Our neonatal thymus transplantation studies and the adult thymus transplantation studies of others suggest a third defect in the BB rat, within the thymus itself, but this defect appears not to be responsible for the development of either the diabetes or the T lymphocytopenia. Rather, the thymic defect appears to control, at least in part, the lymphocyte hyporesponsiveness characteristic of the diabetes-prone BB rat. The role of the RT6 T-cell differentiation antigen in the etiopathogenesis of diabetes in this animal model remains unclear.

References

Abdou NL, Alavi JB, Abdou NI (1976) Human bone marrow lymphocytes: B and T cell precursors and subpopulations. Blood 47: 423–430

Bellgrau D, Naji A, Silvers WK, Markmann JF, Barker CF (1982) Spontaneous diabetes in BB rats: evidence for a T-cell dependent immune response defect. Diabetologia 23: 359–364

Brideau RJ, Carter PB, McMaster WR, Mason DW, Williams AF (1980) Two subsets of rat T lymphocytes defined with monoclonal antibodies. Eur J Immunol 10: 609–615

Burstein D, Mordes JP, Greiner DL, Stein D, Nakamura N, Handler ES, Rossini AA (1989) Prevention of diabetes in BB/Wor rat by single transfusion of spleen cells. Parameters that affect degree of protection. Diabetes 36: 24–30

Cantrell DA, Robins RA, Brooks CG, Baldwin RW (1982) Phenotype of rat natural killer cells defined by monoclonal antibodies marking rat lymphocyte subsets. Immunology 45: 97–103

Colle E, Guttmann RD, Seemayer T (1981) Spontaneous diabetes mellitus syndrome in the rat. I. Association with the major histocompatibility complex. J Exp Med 154: 1237–1242

Dean BM, Bone AJ, Varey AM, Walker R, Baird JD, Cooke A (1987) Insulin autoantibodies, islet cell surface antibodies and the development of spontaneous diabetes in the BB/Edinburgh rat. Clin Exp Immunol 69: 308–313

Dyrberg T, Nakhooda AF, Baekkeskov S, Lernmark Å, Poussier P, Marliss EB (1982) Islet cell surface antibodies and lymphocyte antibodies in the spontaneously diabetic BB Wistar rat. Diabetes 31: 278–281

Elder ME, Maclaren NK (1983) Identification of profound peripheral T lymphocyte immunodeficiencies in the spontaneously diabetic BB rat. J Immunol 130: 1723–1731

Elder M, Maclaren N, Riley W, McConnell T (1982) Gastric parietal cell and other autoantibodies in the BB rat. Diabetes 31: 313–318

Ely JM, Greiner DL, Lubaroff DM, Fitch FW (1983) Characterization of monoclonal antibodies that define rat T cell alloantigens. J Immunol 130: 2798–2803

Fauci AS (1975) Human bone marrow lymphocytes. I. Distribution of lymphocyte subpopulations in the bone marrow of normal individuals. J Clin Invest 56: 98–110

Francfort JW, Naji A, Silvers WK, Barker CF (1985) The influence of T-lymphocyte precursor cells and thymus grafts on the cellular immunodeficiencies of the BB rat. Diabetes 34: 1134–1138

Georgiou HM, Lagarde AC, Bellgrau D (1988) T cell dysfunction in the diabetes-prone BB rat. A role for thymic migrants that are not T cell precursors. J Exp Med 167: 132–148

Greiner DL, Handler ES, Nakano K, Mordes JP, Rossini AA (1986) Absence of RT-6 T cell subset in diabetes-prone BB/W rats. J Immunol 136: 148–151

Greiner DL, Mordes JP, Handler ES, Angellino M, Nakamura N, Rossini AA (1987) Depletion of $RT6.1^+$ T lymphocytes induces diabetes in resistant BioBreeding/Worcester (BB/W) rats. J Exp Med 166: 461–475

Häas RJ, Bohne F, Fliedner TM (1969) On the development of slowly-turning-over cell types in neonatal rat bone marrow. Studies utilizing the complete tritiated thymidine labeling method complemented by C-14 thymidine administration. Blood 34: 791–805

Jackson R, Rassi N, Crump T, Haynes B, Eisenbarth GS (1981) The BB diabetic rat. Profound T-cell lymphocytopenia. Diabetes 30: 887–889

Jackson R, Kadison P, Buse J, Rassi N, Jegasothy B, Eisenbarth GS (1983) Lymphocyte abnormalities in the BB rat. Metabolism 32 [Suppl 1]: 83–86

Jackson RA, Buse JB, Rifai R, Pelletier D, Milford EL, Carpenter CB, Eisenbarth GS, Williams RM (1984) Two genes required for diabetes in BB rats. Evidence from cyclical intercrosses and backcrosses. J Exp Med 159: 1629–1636

Klöting I, Vogt L, Stark O, Fischer U (1987) Genetic heterogeneity in different BB rat subpopulations. Diabetes Res 6: 145–149

Koevary S, Rossini AA, Stoller W, Chick W, Williams RM (1983) Passive transfer of diabetes in the BB/W rat. Science 220: 727–728

Koevary S, Williams DE, Williams RM, Stoller W, Chick WL (1985) Passive transfer of diabetes from BB/W to Wistar-Furth rats. J Clin Invest 75: 1904–1907

Like AA, Rossini AA (1984) Spontaneous autoimmune diabetes mellitus in the Bio-Breeding/Worcester rat. Surv Synth Pathol Res 3: 131–138

Like AA, Rossini AA, Appel MC, Guberski DL, Williams RM (1979) Spontaneous diabetes mellitus: reversal and prevention in the BB/W rat with antiserum to rat lymphocytes. Science 206: 1421–1423

Like AA, Butler L, Williams RM, Appel MC, Weringer EJ, Rossini AA (1982a) Spontaneous autoimmune diabetes mellitus in the BB rat. Diabetes 31[Suppl 1]: 7–13

Like AA, Kislauskis E, Williams RM, Rossini AA (1982b) Neonatal thymectomy prevents spontaneous diabetes mellitus in the BB/W rat. Science 216: 644–646

Like AA, Anthony M, Guberski DL, Rossini AA (1982c) Spontaneous diabetes mellitus in the BB/W rat. Effects of glucocortocoids, cyclosporin-A, and antiserum to rat lymphocytes. Diabetes 32: 326–330

Like AA, Weringer EJ, Holdash A, McGill P, Rossini AA (1985) Adoptive transfer of autoimmune diabetes in BioBreeding/Worcester (BB/W) inbred and hybrid rats. J Immunol 134: 1582–1587

Like AA, Biron CA, Weringer ES, Brayman K, Sroczynski E, Guberski DL (1986) Prevention of diabetes in BioBreeding Worcester rats with monoclonal antibodies that recognize T-lymphocytes or natural killer cells. J Exp Med 164: 1145–1159

Marliss EB, Nakhooda AF, Poussier P, Sima AF (1982) The diabetic syndrome of the 'BB' Wistar rat: Possible relevance to Type 1 (insulin-dependent) diabetes in man. Diabetologia 22: 225–232

Mojcik CF, Greiner DL, Medlock ES, Komschlies KL, Goldschneider I (1988) Characterization of RT6 bearing rat lymphocytes. I. Ontogeny of the $RT6^+$ subset. Cell Immunol 114: 336–346

Mordes JP, Gallina DL, Handler ES, Greiner DL, Nakamura N, Pelletier A, Rossini AA (1987) Transfusions enriched for $W3/25^+$ helper/inducer T lymphocytes prevent spontaneous diabetes in the BB/W rat. Diabetologia 30: 22–26

Naji A, Silvers WK, Bellgrau D, Anderson AO, Plotkin S, Barker CF (1981a) Prevention of diabetes in rats by bone marrow transplantation. Ann Surg 194: 328–338

Naji A, Silvers WK, Bellgrau D, Barker CF (1981b) Spontaneous diabetes in rats: destruction of islets is prevented by immunologic tolerance. Science 213: 1390–1392

Naji A, Bellgrau D, Anderson AO, Silvers WK, Barker CF (1982) Transplantation of islets and bone marrow cells to animals with immune insulitis. Diabetes 31 [Suppl 4]: 84–91

Naji A, Silver WK, Kimura H, Bellgrau D, Markham JF, Barker CF (1983) Analytical and functional studies on the T cells of untreated and immunologically tolerant diabetes-prone BB rats. J Immunol 130: 2168–2172

Nakano K, Mordes JP, Handler ES, Greiner DL, Rossini AA (1988) Role of host immune system in BB/Wor rat. Predisposition to diabetes resides in bone marrow. Diabetes 520–525

Nakhooda AF, Like AA, Chappel CI, Murray FT, Marliss EB (1977) The spontaneously diabetic Wistar rat. Metabolic and morphologic studies. Diabetes 26: 100–112

O'Brien S (Ed.) (1987) In: Genetic maps, vol 4. A compilation of linkage and reconstruction maps of genetically studied organisms. Cold Spring Harbor Laboratory, New York

Poussier P, Nakhooda AF, Falk JA, Lee C, Marliss EB (1982) Lymphopenia and abnormal lymphocyte subsets in the 'BB' rat: relationship to the diabetic syndrome. Endocrinology 110: 1825–1827

Prud'homme GJ, Fuks A, Colle E, Seemayer TA, Guttmann RD (1984) Immune dysfunction in diabetes-prone BB rats. IL-2 production and other mitogen-induced reponses are suppressed by activated macrophages. J Exp Med 463–478

Rossini AA, Williams RM, Mordes JP, Appel MC, Like AA (1979) Spontaneous diabetes in the gnotobiotic BB/W rat. Diabetes 28: 1031–1032

Rossini AA, Mordes JP, Pelletier AM, Like AA (1983) Transfusions of whole blood prevent spontaneous diabetes mellitus in the BB/W rat. Science 219: 975–977

Rossini AA, Mordes JP, Greiner DL, Nakano K, Appel MC, Handler ES (1986) Spleen cell transfusion in the BB/W rat: prevention of diabetes, MHC restriction, and long-term persistence of transfused cells. J Clin Invest 77: 1399–1401

Scott J, Engelhard VH, Benjamin DC (1984) Enhancement of mixed lymphocyte response (MLR) and mitogen stimulation in BB rat lymphocytes by IL-2 (interleukin-2). Diabetes 33[Suppl 1]: 61A (Abstract)

Scott J, Benjamin DC, McGill P, Engelhard VH (1986a) Thymus transplantation with and without prior thymectomy, in neonatal BB/Ch rats. Diabetes 35[Suppl 1]: 69A (Abstract)

Scott J, Engelhard VH, Curnow RT, Benjamin DC (1986b) Prevention of diabetes in BB rats. 1. Evidence suggesting a requirement for mature T cells in bone marrow inoculum of neonatally injected rats. Diabetes 35: 1034–1040

Scott J, Benjamin DC, Scott CA, Herr JC, Engelhard VH (1987a) Effects of neonatal transplantation of MHC-compatible thymuses into diabetes-prone BB rats. Diabetes 36[Suppl 1]: 65A (Abstract)

Scott J, Engelhard VH, Benjamin DC (1987b) Bone marrow irradiation chimeras in the BB rat: evidence suggesting two defects leading to diabetes and lymphopoenia. Diabetologia 30: 774–781

Scott J, Benjamin DC, Herr JC, Engelhard VH (1989) Sites of the defects leading to autoimmunity in the spontaneously diabetic BB rat. In Camerini-Davalos RS (ed) Prediabetes: proceedings of the fifth international symposium on early diabetes. Plenum, New York, pp 53–62

Thiele HG, Koch F, Kashan A (1987) Postnatal distribution profiles of Thy-1^+ and $RT6^+$ cells in peripheral lymph nodes of DA rats. Transplant Proc 19: 3157–3160

Varey AM, Dean BM, Walker R, Bone AJ, Baird JD, Cooke A (1987) Immunological responses of the BB rat colony in Edinburgh. Immunology 60: 131–134

Woda BA, Biron CA (1986) Natural killer cell number and function in the spontaneously diabetic BB/W rat. J Immunol 137: 1860–1866
Woda BA, Like AA, Padden C, McFadden M (1986) Deficiency of phenotypic cytotoxic-suppressor T lymphocytes in the BB/W rat. J Immunol 136: 856–859
Yale JF, Marliss EB (1984) Review. Altered immunity and diabetes in the BB rat. Clin Exp Immunol 57: 1–11

Immune Pathogenesis of Diabetes in the Nonobese Diabetic Mouse: An Overview

T. Hanafusa and S. Tarui

1 Introduction

A considerable amount of evidence suggests that human type 1 or insulin-dependent diabetes mellitus (IDDM) is a chronic autoimmune disease with a long preclinical period. It is extremely difficult to study the process of pancreatic beta cell damage during the preclinical stage of the disease, and only detailed analysis of animal models appears to give us some answers in this important area. In 1974 a female mouse in the normoglycemic subline of Jcl-ICR mice was found to show overt diabetes, and the nonobese diabetic (NOD) mouse strain was subsequently established in the Shionogi Laboratories (Tochino 1986). These mice have many characteristics similar to human type 1 diabetic patients and have been increasingly used as an animal model for type 1 diabetes (Tarui and Hanafusa 1988). This review summarizes the current knowledge on the immune pathogenesis of diabetes in NOD mice.

2 Genetics

Diabetes in the NOD mouse is histologically characterized by the infiltration of lymphocytes into the pancreatic islets (insulitis). Insulitis starts around 4 weeks of age, long before the clinical onset of diabetic symptoms, which start around 15 weeks of age. The occurrence of insulitis and/or diabetic syndrome of the NOD mouse is under genetic control. Makino et al. (1980) reported that the incidence of insulitis is controlled by two recessive genes after crossing NOD mice with C57BL/6J. Hattori et al. (1986) showed by crossing NOD mice with C3H mice that at least three genes are involved in the development of insulitis and diabetes. A similar result was obtained by Prochazka et al. (1987) who also indicated the participation of three recessive genes in the development of diabetes in NOD mice. One of the three diabetogenic genes was found to be linked to the major

The Second Department of Internal Medicine, Osaka University Medical School, Osaka, Japan

Current Topics in Microbiology and Immunology, Vol. 156

histocompatibility complex (MHC) genes on chromosome 17 (Hattori et al. 1986; Prochazka et al. 1987). Interestingly, Wicker et al. (1987) reported that insulitis was controlled by a single incompletely dominant gene, however, the diabetes was controlled by at least three functionally recessive diabetogenic genes, or gene complexes, one of which is linked to the MHC.

The study by Hattori et al. (1986) and the sequence analysis by Acha-Orbea and McDevitt (1987) of the MHC genes and their corresponding molecules have shown that NOD mice have unique MHC properties. First, the I-E_α gene is present, but messenger RNA for Eα is absent, resulting in lack of expression of I-Eα molecules. This property is not entirely restricted to NOD mice, but is found in some other strains of mice such as C57BL. Second, the nucleotide sequence of the A_β gene of NOD mice is different from any known A_β gene, resulting in the expression of a unique A_β molecule. These observations raise the question as to whether these genes are directly responsible for the development of insulitis and/or diabetes in NOD mice.

Nishimoto et al. (1987) studied the participation of the E_α defect in the occurrence of insulitis. After obtaining F1 mice by crossing E_α deficient NOD mice with C57BL mice which had previously been induced by the transgene technique to express the I-E_α molecule, Nishimoto et al. (1987) showed that the expression of I-E_α molecules in $F_1 \times$ NOD backcross mice could prevent the development of autoimmune insulitis. Their most recent transgene experiment with direct injection of the E_α gene into NOD mice has shown that NOD mice induced to express I-E molecules have no sign of insulitis, further suggesting the important role that the E_α defect plays in the occurrence of insulitis.

Another interesting result came from the sequence analysis of human MHC genes. Todd et al. (1987) reported that the HLA-DQ_β gene (human counterpart of mouse I-A_β) contributes to the IDDM susceptibility in humans. They suggested that the aspartic acid (Asp) in residue 57 of the DQ_β chain contributes to the protection of the insulin-producing islet cells against an autoimmune response. The substitution of Asp at this position by other amino acids, such as Ala, Val, or Ser, is found in most IDDM-susceptible haplotypes. The same phenomenon applies to the amino acid sequence of NOD mice, in which position 57 in the I-A_β molecule is Ser, while nondiabetic B10 mice have Asp in this position. The substitution of Asp by other amino acids may alter the three-dimensional configuration of the DQ_β or I-A_β molecules. This may result in the aberrant recognition of islet cell autoantigens by T lymphocytes which finally leads to the development of an autoimmune reaction against the beta cells. Concerning IDDM in humans, it remains to be clarified whether this amino acid substitution occurs in other races than Caucasians.

These results could indicate that either the lack of E_α expression or the unique amino acid sequence of the A_β chain is responsible for the development of diabetes in the NOD mouse. Prochazka et al. (1987) and Ikegami et al. (1986) suggested that a second diabetogenic gene is located near the gene for the T-cell surface antigen, Thy-1, on chromosome 9, however, the precise chromosomal localization of this gene is still uncertain (H. Ikegami and M. Hattori, personal communication). This second gene might play a primary role in the development of insulitis, and the MHC-linked gene might contribute to the progression from insulitis to overt diabetes. No information is available at present on the third diabetogenic gene. Hopefully, the studies employing molecular biological techniques will clarify the role of MHC and other genes in the pathogenesis of diabetes in the NOD mouse as well as in humans.

3 Immunopathogenesis

The participation of autoimmunity in the pathogenesis of insulitis and diabetes in NOD mice has been shown in many studies. The precise identification of the lymphocytes which infiltrate the islets would be the first step in clarifying the autoimmune process which causes the destruction of the pancreatic beta cells. Immunohistochemical analysis by MIYAZAKI et al. (1985) of infiltrating cells has demonstrated that T lymphocytes, especially Lytl or L3T4 T cells, are the main phenotype, at least in the early stage of insulitis. There are relatively few Lyt2 T cells and B lymphocytes start to increase around the T-cell cluster in the later stage of the insulitis. Asialo-GM1-positive natural killer (NK) cells are seen in some islets. This finding suggests an important role for L3T4 T cells in the initiation of insulitis. However, it is still necessary to directly demonstrate this subset so as to establish its exact role in insulitis. The crucial question is: Can insulitis be transferred with L3T4 T-cells?

Several attempts have been made to transfer insulitis with spleen cells of NOD mice. WICKER et al. (1986) first showed that diabetes was inducible in irradiated NOD mice by injecting splenocytes from donor NOD mice. The lymphocyte subset responsible for the transfer of insulitis or diabetes was then studied in several laboratories, including our own. HARADA (1987) reported the successful induction of insulitis, but not of diabetes, in athymic NOD nude recipients by transferring thymocytes or splenocytes from euthymic littermates. To study the role of T lymphocytes, especially Lytl or L3T4 T cells, in the pathogenesis of insulitis, we employed T lymphocyte-depleted NOD mice (NOD B mice) as the recipient and performed a transfer study (HANAFUSA et al. 1988). After confirming that these mice rarely develop insulitis, splenic lymphocytes from cyclophosphamide-treated donor NOD mice were fractionated using various monoclonal antibodies against different T-cell surface markers and injected into the recipient NOD B mice. Histological examination 2 weeks after the cell transfer revealed that the Lyt2 T lymphocyte-depleted fraction, which contains L3T4 cells, successfully induced insulitis in the recipient mice. However, the L3T4 T cell-depleted fraction, which contains Lyt2 cells, was unable to transfer insulitis indicating that L3T4 T lymphocytes are a necessary component for the transfer of insulitis in NOD mice. This finding is consistent with other reports, which include studies dealing with the prevention of insulitis and diabetes.

KOIKE et al. (1987) reported the successful prevention of insulitis in NOD mice treated with anti-L3T4 monoclonal antibodies. The same effect of this antibody was also reported by CHARLTON and MANDEL (1988) in cyclophosphamide-induced diabetes. A similar result was obtained by WANG et al. (1987), who found that anti-L3T4 treatment in NOD mice prevented the destruction of grafted BALB/c islets. MILLER et al. (1988) and BENDELAC et al. (1987) suggested that L3T4 T cells could induce insulitis, but this subset alone was not sufficient to induce diabetes. Their experiments indicated that Lyt2 cells were required for the progression from insulitis to overt diabetes. $Lyt2^{+}$ T lymphocytes were shown by TIMSIT et al. (1988) to inhibit insulin release from normal islet cells in response to theophylline plus arginine. HASKINS et al. (1988) recently cloned from an NOD mouse a $CD4^{+}$ ($L3T4^{+}$) T-cell line which proliferates and produces lymphokine in response to islet cell antigen- and NOD antigen-presenting cells. This cell line was shown to destroy grafted islet cells in a tissue-specific manner. TERADA et al. (1988) suggested that anti-islet immunity in diabetic NOD mice exerts its effect in an H-2-restricted manner. From these studies, it could be postulated that L3T4 T cells initiate insulitis and thereafter help Lyt2 T cells destroy insulin-producing beta cells in a tissue-specific and H-2-restricted manner. Lyt2 cells possibly impair insulin secretion from beta cells. Alternatively, a fraction of $L3T4^{+}$ cells might exhibit cytotoxicity against islet cells.

That macrophages are involved in the occurrence of insulitis or diabetes has recently been suggested by several authors (LEE et al. 1988; CHARLTON et al. 1988) who showed the preventive effect of silica in cyclophosphamide-induced diabetes of NOD mice. The importance of abnormal suppressor cell function has also been reported in several publications. After examining the syngeneic mixed lymphocyte reaction (SMLR), a T-cell response to self-MHC class II antigens, SERREZE and LEITER (1988) found a defect in suppressor cell activation rather than the absence of this immunoregulatory cell population in NOD mice. YASUNAMI and BACH (1988) found that spleen T cells from cyclophosphamide (CY)-induced diabetic NOD mice were capable of transferring the disease into irradiated nondiabetic syngeneic recipients. They found that the diabetogenic effect of CY was mediated by abrogation of a suppressor mechanism which may have prevented the activation of the T cells responsible for the development of diabetes in the NOD mouse. Other immune reactions such as antibody-dependent cell-mediated cytotoxicity (ADCC) may be involved in the beta-cell destruction in NOD mice. NAKAJIMA et al. (1986) has reported that the nonspecific ADCC activity of NOD mice is increased. However, the importance of this phenomenon in the pathogenesis of diabetes in NOD mice remains to be seen.

Then, where do these immunological abnormalities originate? IKEHARA et al. (1985) reported that insulitis of 6-month-old NOD mice was abolished by the reconstitution with bone marrow cells from young BALB/c nu/nu mice, suggesting a role of the bone marrow stem cells. A similar result was reported by WICKER et al. (1988) who showed, by constructing radiation bone marrow chimeras between NOD and B10 mice, that the expression of the diabetic phenotype in NOD mice is dependent on the presence of NOD-derived hematopoietic stem cells. SERREZE et al. (1988a) found that autoimmune beta-cell destruction occurred in otherwise diabetes-resistant F1 mice from an outcross between the NOD and nonobese normal (NON) strains after the adoptive transfer of hematopoietic stem cells from NOD donors. Taken together, these data suggest the presence of abnormal hematopoietic stem cells in the bone marrow of NOD mice.

As for humoral immunity, the presence of various autoantibodies has been reported in the sera of NOD mice. REDDY et al. (1988) reported that islet cell antibodies (ICA) and insulin autoantibodies (IAA) were present at day 15 in about 50% of NOD mice and that the incidence of ICA ranged around 50% from day 25–90, while IAA was detected in all samples during this period. We have also found ICA in NOD mice, but less frequently. The prevalence of ICA in our study was 17%, 33%, 25%, and 17% at 9, 14, 20, and 42 weeks respectively (HANAFUSA et al. 1989). The highest prevalence was observed at 14 weeks, just before diabetic symptoms started. PONTESILLI et al. (1987) reported the presence of autoantibodies likely to be IAA, reacting with the cytoplasm of islet cells in Bouin's fixed pancreas sections in 47%–58% of the samples from NOD mice aged 75–150 days. IAA were detected by enzyme-linked immunoadsorbent assay (ELISA) in all the NOD mice studied. MARUYAMA et al. (1988) also showed the appearance of IAA in 8 out of 9 female and 9 out of 20 male NOD mice.

The presence of antibodies which react with the surface of islet cells (ICSA) has been reported by several laboratories although with different incidences. YOKONO et al. (1984) first established the monoclonal ICSA from NOD splenocytes. This monoclonal antibody exhibited ADCC activity, but not complement-dependent antibody-mediated cytotoxicity (CAMC) (HARI et al. 1986). More recently, autoantibodies reacting with a M_r 64000 beta-cell protein have been detected in NOD mice (ATKINSON and MACLAREN 1988). The autoantibody was detectable by weaning, but disappeared within weeks after the onset of diabetes and was absent in older nondiabetic NOD mice.

Other autoantibodies have also been reported in NOD mice (HANAFUSA et al. 1989) e.g., reacting with the apical border of the thyroid follicular cells or with the duct cells of submandibular glands. Old NOD mice had antinuclear antibodies. However, sera from NOD mice did not contain antibodies against adrenal glands or gastric parietal cells regardless of age.

Since class II MHC antigens were detected on the thyroid follicular cells in patients with Graves' disease and Hashimoto's thyroiditis (HANAFUSA et al. 1983), endocrine cells expressing class II molecules have been hypothesized to present their autoantigens to helper T cells, thus initiating autoimmune reactions against the endocrine cells (BOTTAZZO et al. 1983). Following this hypothesis, several reports appeared on the ectopic expression of class II MHC antigens in organ-specific autoimmune diseases, including type 1 diabetes. The expression of class II molecules on beta cells in type 1 diabetes has been reported in pancreas autopsy samples from newly diagnosed type 1 diabetic patients (BOTTAZZO et al. 1985; FOULIS and FARGUHARSON 1986). In NOD mice, however, controversial results have been reported on this issue using different systems (HANAFUSA et al. 1987; SIGNORE et al. 1987). Further studies are thus necessary on this subject.

4 Viruses and Diabetes in NOD Mice

Viruses have been implicated in the pathogenesis of type 1 diabetes in both humans and animals, and it would therefore be of interest to investigate whether viruses are involved in the destruction of beta cells in NOD mice. Our group has first demonstrated the presence of retrovirus-like particles in NOD mouse islet cells (FUJITA et al. 1984; FUJINO-KURIHARA et al. 1985). The particles were observed exclusively in beta cells of the NOD mouse pancreas. Other endocrine cells such as alpha cells, delta cells, and exocrine acinar cells did not contain such particles. The particles were even detected in 18-day-old fetal NOD mice. The number of retrovirus-like particles increased with age, and about 5% of beta cells contained the particles at around 8 weeks age, when insulitis is most prominent. The particles then became difficult to observe since the progression of beta cells themselves. The presence of retrovirus-like particles was confirmed by SUENAGA and YOON (1988). who frequently found the particles in the beta cells of NOD mice treated with CY. This drug is known to induce diabetes in the relatively diabetes-resistant male NOD mice and it would be interesting to know whether the induction of diabetes is related to the activation of endogenous retroviruses in beta cells. Further, SERREZE et al. (1988b) showed molecular mimicry between insulin and retroviral antigen p73 by detecting cross-reactive autoantibodies in sera of NOD mice.

It should be noted that, although endogenous retroviruses may be involved in the pathogenesis of beta-cell destruction in NOD mice, infection of NOD mice with an exogenous virus may reduce the incidence of diabetes. OLDSTONE (1988) reported that when newborn or adult NOD mice were infected with a lymphotropic virus, they did not become diabetic. Furthermore, lymphocytes from virus-infected donors failed to transfer diabetes, suggesting that the interaction between viruses and lymphocytes is pivotal in aborting diabetes. Interestingly, a similar phenomenon was observed in the BB rat (DYRBERG et al. 1988), another animal model for type 1 diabetes. It is possible that infection with an exogenous virus modulates the preexisting autoimmune responses to beta cells, thereby decreasing the immunological attack against the cells and ameliorating the development of diabetes. The precise mechanisms for this interesting phenomenon remains to be clarified.

5 Immunomodulation

Various attempts have been made to prevent insulitis and/or diabetes in NOD mice (HANAFUSA and TARUI 1989). Many of them are related to the modulation of the immune system. In this overview, we would like to discuss areas which are relevant to the pathogenesis of diabetes in NOD mice.

Neonatal thymectomy has been shown to prevent the occurrence of diabetes in NOD mice, further supporting the participation of T lymphocytes in the development of diabetes (OGAWA et al. 1985). Cyclosporine (CS) is a potent immunosuppressive agent. This drug seems to derive its action from inhibition of the release of interleukin-1 and interleukin-2 (IL-1, IL-2), both of which are involved in the generation of helper T cells. KIDA et al. (1986) showed that the oral administration of 20 or 40 mg/kg per day of CS for 5 weeks from the age of 4 weeks reduced the incidence of insulitis. CS suppressed insulitis more markedly in male than in female mice. MORI et al. (1986) showed that a lower dose of CS (2.5 mg/kg every 2 days) was enough to prevent diabetes, and none of the mice developed diabetes even after cessation of CS. Histologic examination revealed that the islets of the mice whose diabetes had been prevented with CS had an almost normal appearance. However, CS treatment of NOD mice which had already developed diabetes (25 mg/kg every 2 days) did not cure the disease. Similar results were reported by WANG et al. (1988), who showed that CS was ineffective in controlling the recurrence of the disease in the islet grafts transplanted to diabetic animals. These results suggest that, although CS has been reported by several laboratories to be beneficial in treating newly diagnosed type 1 diabetic patients, the treatment should preferably be started before onset of the disease. A different regimen for CS immunosuppression was investigated by FORMBY et al. (1988), who showed that autologous spleen lymphocytes from 12-week-old nondiabetic female NOD mice cultured for 72 h with CS and IL-2 lost their ability to induce diabetes in the recipient mice. The authors suggested an ex vivo preferential IL-2 activation of specific suppressor cells for the autoimmune process with CS blockade of cytolytic/helper activities.

Nicotinamide is a precursor for nicotinamide adenine dinucleotide (NAD) and a potent inhibitor of poly(ADP-ribose) synthetase and other ADP-ribosyltransferase. We examined the effect of nicotinamide on spontaneously occurring diabetes in NOD mice, since the administration of nicotinamide has been reported not only to prevent diabetes produced with a single administration of streptozotocin (STZ) but to attenuate insulitis induced by multiple small dose STZ injections (YAMADA et al. 1982). Daily subcutaneous injections of nicotinamide at a dose of 0.5 mg/g body weight for at least 40 days prevented the development of diabetes in female NOD mice. The islets of the mice treated with nicotinamide were relatively preserved and had only mild insulitis. Nicotinamide had not only preventive, but therapeutic effects in NOD mice. When the nicotinamide injections was started from the day of the first appearance of marked glycosuria, more than half of the mice became aglycosuric within 3 weeks and showed almost normal glucose tolerance after nicotinamide treatment for 40 days. Nicotinamide was effective in ameliorating lymphocytic infiltration into submandibular glands but had no effect on the prevalence of antisubmandibular gland duct cell antibodies. This agent also prevented CY-induced diabetes in NOD mice when the daily nicotinamide treatment was started on the day of the CY injection (NAKAJIMA et al. 1985). The combined treatment of the mice with nicotinamide and desferrioxamine, an iron chelator and inhibitor of hydroxy radical formation, prevented the destruction of transplanted BALB/c islets (NOMIKOS et al. 1986). The animals with transplants became normoglycemic and remained so for the duration of treatment.

The mechanism of nicotinamide action could be postulated as follows. First, nicotinamide has been shown to inhibit ADCC activity (NAKAJIMA et al. 1986) and thus may modulate immune responses. Second, nicotinamide might be utilized to produce NAD, which might be reduced in islets of NOD mice. Alternatively, nicotinamide may act as an inhibitor of poly(ADP-ribose) synthetase (UCHIGATA et al. 1982), thus preventing the reduction of NAD and the breakdown of DNA at the same time. It requires further careful evaluation to establish whether nicotinamide is effective in treating human type 1 diabetes.

Although the incidence of insulitis is almost the same between male and female NOD mice, a marked sex difference in the incidence of diabetes has been observed. This suggests that sex hormones modulate the development of diabetes from insulitis. Several attempts have been made to modulate the occurrence of diabetes with sex hormones. MAKINO et al. (1981) performed ovariectomy and orchiectomy on 5-week-old NOD mice. The cumulative incidence of diabetes in castrated NOD male mice was similar to that of nonoperated female mice. Conversely, females with ovariectomy showed a low incidence of overt diabetes equal to that in males. A similar experiment by TOCHINO (unpublished observation) showed that the removal of sex organs at 10 weeks of age did not affect the incidence of diabetes in either sex. However, when testosterone was administered to these mice, no animals from either sex developed diabetes, while when estradiol was given, overt diabetes appeared in mice of both sexes. These results directly demonstrate that sex hormones regulate the development of diabetes in NOD mice. It would be interesting to know the effects of sex hormones on the immunological responses.

Diet was also shown by ELLIOTT et al. (1988) to affect the incidence of diabetes in NOD mice. Only mice receiving meat or casein as the source of protein developed diabetes, whereas lactalbumin and gluten did not precipitate diabetes except in a small number of mice. Casein hydrolysate in lieu of protein protected against overt diabetes. However, the mice had intermittent trace glycosuria, and the majority showed mild degrees of peri-insular lymphocytic infiltration. The mechanism of the diet's preventive effect remains to be seen, and how it relates to human IDDM is still unclear.

6 Conclusion

Vast amounts of data have been reported since the discovery and establishment of the NOD mouse strain, especially in the past few years. The striking similarities between the diabetic syndrome of the NOD mouse and human IDDM has led to the extensive use of these animals in the study of IDDM. However, it should be borne in mind that IDDM patients are both genetically and probably pathogenically heterogeneous and thus NOD mice may only be representative of part of the population of IDDM patients. It is also possible that the pathogenic mechanism by which the beta cells are destroyed in NOD mice is considerably different from that in IDDM patients. Nevertheless, the NOD mouse is an indispensable model, and it will continue to give us important clues to the pathogenesis and the treatment of human IDDM. We believe that by taking full advantage of an animal model, and not being discouraged by its disadvantages, we can reach the final goal–preventing and treating human IDDM.

References

Acha-Orbea H, McDevitt HO (1987) The first external domain of the nonobese diabetic mouse class II I-A chain is unique. Proc Natl Acad Sci USA 84: 2435–2439

Atkinson MA, Maclaren NK (1988) Autoantibodies in nonobese diabetic mice immunoprecipitate 64,000-M(r) islet antigen. Diabetes 37: 1587–1590

Bendelac A, Carnaud C, Boitard C, Bach JF (1987) Syngeneic transfer of autoimmune diabetes from diabetic NOD mice to healthy neonates. Requirement for both $L3T4^+$ and $Lyt2^+$ cells. J Exp Med 166: 823–832

Bottazzo GF, Pujol-Borrell R, Hanafusa T, Feldmann M (1983) Role of aberrant HLA-DR expression and antigen presentation in the induction of endocrine autoimmunity. Lancet 2: 1115–1119

Bottazzo GF, Dean BM, McNally JM, Mackay EH, Swift PGF, Gamble DR (1985) In situ characterization of autoimmune phenomena and expression of HLA molecules in the pancreas in diabetic insulitis. N Engl J Med 313: 353–360

Charlton B, Mandel TE (1988) Progression from insulitis to beta-cell destruction in NOD mouse requires $L3T4^+$ T-lymphocytes. Diabetes 37: 1108–1112

Charlton B, Bacelj A, Mandel TE (1988) Administration of silica particles or anti-Lyt2 antibody prevents beta-cell destruction in NOD mice given cyclophosphamide. Diabetes 37: 930–935

Dyrberg T, Schwimmbeck PL, Oldstone MBA (1988) Inhibition of diabetes in BB rats by virus infection. J Clin Invest 81: 928–931

Elliott RB, Reddy SN, Bibby NJ, Kida K (1988) Dietary prevention of diabetes in the non-obese diabetic mouse. Diabetologia 31: 62–64

Formby B, Miller N, Peterson CM (1988) Adoptive immunotherapy of diabetes in autologous nonobese diabetic mice with lymphoid cells ex vivo exposed to cyclosporin plus interleukin 2. Diabetes 37: 1305–1309

Foulis AK, Farquharson MA (1986) Aberrant expression of HLA-DR antigens by insulin containing beta-cells in recent-onset Type I diabetes mellitus. Diabetes 35: 1215–1224

Fujino-Kurihara H, Fujita H, Hakura A, Nonaka K, Tarui S (1985) Morphological aspects on pancreatic islets of nonobese diabetic (NOD) mice. Virchows Arch B [Cell Pathol] 49: 107–120

Fujita H, Fujino H, Nonaka K, Tarui S, Tochino Y (1984) Retrovirus-like particles in pancreatic B-cells of NOD (nonobese diabetic) mice. Biomed Res 5: 67–70

Hanafusa T, Tarui S (1989) Immunotherapy of the NOD mouse. In: Eisenbarth GS (ed) Immunotherapy of diabetes and selected autoimmune diseases. CRC Press, Boca Raton, Florida, pp 53–60

Hanafusa T, Pujol-Borrell R, Chiovato L, Russell RCG, Doniach D, Bottazzo GF (1983) Aberrant expression of HLA-DR antigen on thyrocytes in Graves' disease: relevance for autoimmunity. Lancet 2: 1111–1115

Hanafusa T, Fujino-Kurihara H, Miyazaki A, Yamada K, Nakajima H, Miyagawa J, Kono N, Tarui S (1987) Expression of class II major histocompatibility complex antigens on pancreatic B cells in the NOD mouse. Diabetologia 30: 104–108

Hanafusa T, Sugihara S, Fujino-Kurihara H, Miyagawa J, Miyazaki A, Yoshioka T, Yamada K, Nakajima H, Asakawa H, Kono N, Fujiwara H, Hamaoka T, Tarui S (1988) The induction of insulitis by adoptive transfer with L3T4$^+$Lyt-2$^-$ T-lymphocytes in T-lymphocyte-depleted NOD mice. Diabetes 37: 204–208

Hanafusa T, Miyazaki A, Yamada K, Miyagawa J, Fujino-Kurihara H, Nakajima H, Kono N, Nonaka K, Tarui S (1988) Autoantibodies to islet cells and multiple organs in the NOD mouse. Diabetes Nutr Metab 1: 273–276

Harada M (1987) Immune disturbance and pathogenesis of non-obese diabetes-prone (NOD) mice. Exp Clin Endocrinol 89: 251–258

Hari J, Yokono K, Yonezawa K, Amano K, Yaso S, Shii K, Imamura Y, Baba S (1986) Immunochemical characterization of anti-islet cell surface monoclonal antibody from nonobese diabetic mice. Diabetes 35: 517–522

Haskins K, Portas M, Bradley B, Wegmann D, Lafferty K (1988) T-lymphocyte clone specific for pancreatic islet antigen. Diabetes 37: 1444–1448

Hattori M, Buse JB, Jackson RA, Glimcher L, Dorf ME, Minami M, Makino, Moriwaki K, Kuzuya H, Imura H, Strauss WM, Seidman JG, Eisenbarth GS (1986) The NOD mouse: recessive diabetogenic gene in the major histocompatibility complex. Science 231: 733–735

Ikegami H, Hattori M, Makino S, Eisenbarth GS (1986) Analysis of the immunogenetics of the NOD mouse utilizing multiple strain combinations: two recessive diabetogenic genes linked with H-2 (chromosome 17) and Thy-1 (chromosome 9). Paper presented at the symposium on the immunology of diabetes, Edmonton, Canada, June 1986 Abstract no S7

Ikehara S, Ohtsuki H, Good RA, Asamoto H, Nakamura T, Sekita K, Muso E, Tochino Y, Ida T, Kuzuya H, Imura H, Hamashima Y (1985) Prevention of type I diabetes in nonobese diabetic mice by allogeneic bone marrow transplantation. Proc Natl Acad Sci USA 82: 7743–7747

Kida K, Kaino Y, Miyagawa T, Gotoh Y, Matsuda H (1986) Effect of cyclosporin on insulitis and ICSA in NOD mice. In: Tarui S, Nonaka K, Tochino Y (eds) Insulitis and Type I diabetes: lessons from animal diabetes. Academic, Tokyo, pp 137–142

Koike T, Itoh Y, Ishii T, Ito I, Takabayashi K, Maruyama N, Tomioka H, Yoshida S (1987) Preventive effect of monoclonal anti-L3T4 antibody on development of diabetes in NOD mice. Diabetes 36: 539–541

Lee K, Amano K, Yoon J (1988) Evidence for initial involvement of macrophage in development of insulitis in NOD mice. Diabetes 37: 989–991

Makino S, Kunimoto K, Muraoka Y, Mizushima Y, Katagiri K, Tochino Y (1980) Breeding of a non-obese diabetic strain of mice. Exp Animals (Tokyo) 29: 1–13

Makino S, Kunimoto K, Muraoka Y, Katagiri K (1981) Effect of castration on the appearance of diabetes in NOD mouse. Exp Anim 30: 137–140

Maruyama T, Takei I, Yanagawa T, Takahashi T, Asaba Y, Kataoka K, Ishii T (1988) Insulin autoantibodies in nonobese diabetic (NOD) mice and streptozotocin-induced diabetic mice. Diabetes Res 7: 93–96

Miller BJ, Appel MC, O'Neil JJ, Wicker LS (1988) Both the Lyt-2$^+$ and L3T4$^+$ T cell subsets are required for the transfer of diabetes in nonobese diabetic mice. J Immunol 140: 52–58

Miyazaki A, Hanafusa T, Yamada K, Miyagawa J, Fujino-Kurihara H, Nakajima H, Nonaka K, Tarui S (1985) Predominance of T lymphocytes in pancreatic islets and spleen of pre-diabetic non-obese diabetic (NOD) mice: a longitudinal study. Clin Exp Immunol 60: 622–630

Mori Y, Suko M, Okudaira H, Matsuba I, Tsuruoka A, Sasaki A, Yokoyama H, Tanase T, Shiba T, Nishimura M, Terada E, Ikeda Y (1986) Preventive effects of cyclosporin on diabetes in NOD mice. Diabetologia 29: 244–247

Nakajima H, Fujino-Kurihara H, Hanafusa T, Yamada K, Miyazaki A, Miyagawa J, Nonaka K, Tarui S, Tochino Y (1985) Nicotinamide prevents the development of cyclophosphamide-induced diabetes mellitus in male non-obese diabetic (NOD) mice. Biomed Res 6: 185–189

Nakajima H, Yamada K, Hanafusa T, Fujino-Kurihara H, Miyagawa J, Miyazaki A, Saitoh R, Minami Y, Kono N, Nonaka K, Tochino Y, Tarui S (1986) Elevated antibody-dependent cell-mediated cytotoxicity and its inhibition by nicotinamide in the diabetic NOD mouse. Immunol Lett 12: 91–94

Nishimoto H, Kikutani H, Yamamura K, Kishimoto T (1987) Prevention of autoimmune insulitis by expression of I-E molecules in NOD mice. Nature 328: 432–434

Nomikos IN, Prowse SJ, Carotenuto P, Lafferty KJ (1986) Combined treatment with nicotinamide and desferrioxamine prevents islet allograft destruction in NOD mice. Diabetes 35: 1302–1304

Ogawa M, Maruyama T, Hasegawa T, Kanaya T, Kobayashi F, Tochino Y, Uda H (1985) The inhibitory effect of neonatal thymectomy on the incidence of insulitis in non-obese diabetes (NOD) mice. Biomed Res 6: 103–105

Oldstone MBA (1988) Prevention of type I diabetes in nonobese diabetic mice by virus infection. Science 239: 500–502

Pontesilli O, Carotenuto P, Gazda LS, Pratt PF, Prowse SJ (1987) Circulating lymphocyte populations and autoantibodies in non-obese diabetic (NOD) mice: a longitudinal study. Clin Exp Immunol 70: 84–93

Prochazka M, Leiter EH, Serreze DV, Coleman DL (1987) Three recessive loci required for insulin-dependent diabetes in nonobese diabetic mice. Science 237: 286–289

Reddy S, Bibby NJ, Elliott RB (1988) Ontogeny of islet cell antibodies, insulin autoantibodies and insulitis in the non-obese diabetic mouse. Diabetologia 31: 322–328

Serreze DV, Leiter EH (1988) Defective activation of T suppressor cell function in nonobese diabetic mice: potential relation to cytokine deficiencies. J Immunol 140: 3801–3807

Serreze DV, Leiter EH, Worthen SM, Shultz LD (1988a) NOD marrow stem cells adoptively transfer diabetes to resistant (NOD × NON)F1 mice. Diabetes 37: 252–255

Serreze DV, Leiter EH, Kuff EL, Jardieu P, Ishizaka K (1988b) Molecular mimicry between insulin and retroviral antigen p73. Development of cross-reactive autoantibodies in sera of NOD and C57BL/KsJ db/db mice. Diabetes 37: 351–358

Signore A, Cooke A, Pozzilli P, Butcher F, Simpson E, Beverley PCL (1987) Class-II and IL2 receptor positive cells in the pancreas of NOD mice. Diabetologia 30: 902–905

Suenaga K, Yoon JW (1988) Association of beta-cell-specific expression of endogenous retrovirus with development of insulitis and diabetes in NOD mouse. Diabetes 37: 1722–1726

Tarui S, Hanafusa T (1988) The NOD mouse. In: Alberti KGMM, Krall LP (eds) The diabetes annual/4. Elsevier, Amsterdam, pp 609–620

Terada M, Salzler M, Lennartz K, Mullen Y (1988) The effect of H-2 compatibility on pancreatic beta cell survival in the nonobese diabetic mouse. Transplantation 45: 622–627

Timsit J, Debray-Sachs M, Boitard C, Bach JF (1988) Cell-mediated immunity to pancreatic islet cells in the non-obese diabetic (NOD) mouse: in vitro characterization and time course study. Clin Exp Immunol 73: 260–264

Tochino Y (1986) Discovery and breeding of the NOD mouse. In: Tarui S, Nonaka K, Tochino Y (eds) Insulitis and Type 1 diabetes: lessons from animal diabetes. Academic, Tokyo, pp 3–10

Todd JA, Bell JI, McDevitt HO (1987) HLA-DQ gene contributes to susceptibility and resistance to insulin-dependent diabetes mellitus. Nature 329: 599–604

Uchigata Y, Yamamoto H, Kawamura A, Okamoto H (1982) Protection by superoxide dismutase, catalase, and poly(ADP-ribose) synthetase inhibitors against alloxan- and streptozotocin-induced islet DNA strand breaks and against the inhibition of proinsulin synthesis. J Biol Chem 257: 6084–6088

Wang Y, Hao L, Gill RG, Lafferty KJ (1987) Autoimmune diabetes in NOD mouse is L3T4 T-lymphocyte dependent. Diabetes 36: 535–538

Wang Y, McDuffie M, Nomikos IN, Hao L, Lafferty KJ (1988) Effect of cyclosporine on immunologically mediated diabetes in nonobese diabetic mice. Transplantation 46[Suppl]: 101S–106S

Wicker LS, Miller BJ, Mullen Y (1986) Transfer of autoimmune diabetes mellitus with splenocytes from nonobese diabetic (NOD) mice. Diabetes 35: 855–860

Wicker LS, Miller BJ, Coker LZ, McNally SE, Scott S, Mullen Y, Appel MC (1987) Genetic control of diabetes and insulitis in the nonobese diabetic (NOD) mouse. J Exp Med 165: 1639–1654

Wicker LS, Miller BJ, Chai A, Terada M, Mullen Y (1988) Expression of genetically determined diabetes and insulitis in the nonobese diabetic (NOD) mouse at the level of bone marrow-derived cells. Transfer of diabetes and insulitis to nondiabetic (NOD × B10)F_1 mice with bone marrow cells from NOD mice. J Exp Med 167: 1801–1810

Yamada K, Nonaka K, Hanafusa T, Miyazaki A, Toyoshima H, Tarui S (1982) Preventive and therapeutic effects of large-dose nicotinamide injections on diabetes associated with insulitis. An observation in nonobese diabetic (NOD) mice. Diabetes 31: 749–753

Yasunami R, Bach JF (1988) Anti-suppressor effect of cyclophosphamide on the development of spontaneous diabetes in NOD mice. Eur J Immunol 18: 481–484

Yokono K, Shii K, Hari J, Yaso S, Imamura Y, Ejiri K, Ishihara K, Fujii S, Kazumi T, Taniguchi H, Baba S (1984) Production of monoclonal antibodies to islet cell surface antigens using hybridization of spleen lymphocytes from non-obese diabetic mice. Diabetologia 26: 379–385

Streptozotocin Interactions with Pancreatic β Cells and the Induction of Insulin-Dependent Diabetes

G. L. WILSON[1] and E. H. LEITER[2]

1 Introduction

The single most consistent finding in insulin-dependent diabetes mellitus (IDDM) is a substantial reduction in insulin secreting β cells (GEPTS 1965). The pathogenic factors responsible for this cellular destruction are complex and most likely differ among different subgroups in this category. Although these factors have not yet been definitively elucidated, it has become apparent that genetic influences and both humoral and cell mediated immunological phenomena are involved (EISENBARTH 1986; LEFEBVRE 1988). Also, a role for environmental factors in the etiology of IDDM has recently been indicated by epidemiological studies which have demonstrated that there is a marked increase in newly diagnosed cases of IDDM, which can only be explained by changes in environmental influences such as chemicals and viruses (KROWLEWSKI et al. 1987). Direct evidence that an ingested chemical can cause IDDM in humans comes from case reports of individuals who ate the rat poison Vacor in suicide attempts. Many of these individuals developed ketosis prone diabetes mellitus (KARAM et al. 1980; PROSSER and KARAM 1978). Studies in laboratory animals have provided additional evidence that xenobiotics can cause a critical reduction in insulin secreting cells. It is well established that nitrosamides like streptozotocin (SZ) and chlorozotocin and other complex amines like alloxan cause severe diabetes in laboratory animals (DULIN and SORET 1977; COOPERSTEIN and WATKINS 1981; MOSSMAN et al. 1985). These and other structurally similar compounds pose a potential threat to humans, either through formation of these agents in the body or through trace contamination in the environment (MAGEE and BARNES 1956; SESFONTEIN and HUSTER 1966; HEDLER and MARQUARDT 1968; SANDER and BURKE 1971; SEN 1973; HAWKSWORTH and HILL 1974; MAGEE 1975; AMES 1983; KNEIP et al. 1983). A correlation between ingested toxins and IDDM has been suggested by epidemiological studies from Iceland. These studies indicated that IDDM developed in some male offspring of mothers who ingested

[1] Department of Structural and Cellular Biology University of South Alabama, Mobile, Alabama 36688

[2] The Jackson Laboratory Bar Harbor, Maine 04609

Current Topics in Microbiology and Immunology, Vol. 156

smoked mutton (Helgason and Jonasson 1981; Helgason et al. 1982). When this meat was analyzed, it was found to contain a significant amount of various *N*-nitroso compounds. However, to date, studies linking these chemicals to the induction of IDDM have been inconclusive.

Until recently, the abrupt onset of clinical symptoms in IDDM had been cited as evidence that there was an environmental component in the etiology of this disease (Craighead 1978). However, the recent discovery that at least some forms of IDDM have a slow progressive pathogenesis has necessitated a conceptual change in how environmental factors may influence the development of this form of IDDM (Eisenbarth 1986). One possibility is that xenobiotics may trigger the onset of autoimmune processes directed toward β cells in genetically susceptible individuals. An alternative possibility would be for toxins to augment the destruction of β cells by the immune system and hasten or precipitate the manifestations of clinical symptoms of IDDM. Studies using the naturally occurring antibiotic streptozotocin have presented direct evidence that xenobiotics may indeed be able to trigger an autoimmune response directed toward β cells. In 1976 Like and Rossini demonstrated that a delayed onset diabetes could be induced in outbred CD-1 mice by giving repeated subdiabetogenic doses of SZ. When the islets from these animals were inspected histologically, an infiltration of mononuclear cells was evident around and throughout the islet. This observation suggested that in addition to the overt toxic effects of SZ, this chemical induced a cell mediated inflammatory response directed against the islets which resulted in further β cell depletion. Also of interest in the islets of these animals was the presence of C type retrovirus. It has been speculated, although not proven, that these particles may be the antigenic trigger for the inflammation (Appel et al. 1978). While the exact pathways by which SZ may alter the β cell to express neoantigens which could elicit an inflammatory response or alter the immune system to precipitate insulitis have yet to be resolved, an understanding of the basic chemistry of this toxin can provide some insights into possible mechanisms.

2 Mechanisms of Action of Streptozotocin

SZ is a naturally occurring antibiotic produced by *Streptomyces achromogenes* (Wiggans et al. 1958). This chemical was originally screened for use in cancer chemotherapy since it had previously been demonstrated that other nitrosoureas had potent anticancer properties. During preclinical screening, SZ was found to be diabetogenic in rats and dogs (Rakieten 1963). Additional experimentation revealed that this chemical produced diabetes in a variety of laboratory animals including mice and guinea pigs (Brosky and Logothetopoulos 1969), hamsters (Wilander and Boquist 1972) and rabbits (Lazarus and Sharpiro 1973). Its structure has been determined to be the nitrosamide methylnitrosourea (MNU)

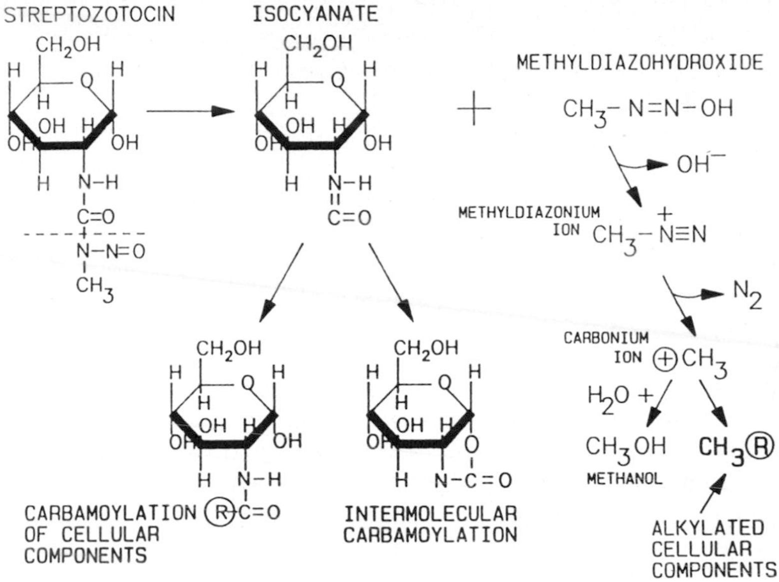

Fig. 1. Spontaneous decomposition of streptozotocin to form carbamoylating and alkylating species

linked to the C-2 position of D-glucose (Fig. 1). The glucose moiety is apparently the essential component in SZ that specifically directs it to the beta cell. Evidence for this is provided by studies which show that MNU is much less toxic to β cells (LEDOUX et al. 1986), and cells that have lost their responsiveness to glucose also lose sensitivity to SZ toxicity (LEDOUX and WILSON 1984). Additionally, studies with SZ labeled with ^{14}C show that considerably more of this toxin is taken up by the β cell than the aglycone MNU (WILSON et al. 1988). If both of these chemicals entered the cell by simple diffusion across the cell membrane, it would be expected that more MNU would be incorporated since it is the smaller molecule. Indeed, this is the finding in RINr cells which are resistant to the toxic effects of SZ (WILSON et al. 1988).

Like most of the nitrosamides, once inside the cell, SZ is able to spontaneously decompose, without metabolizing, to form an isocyanate compound and a methyldiazohydroxide (TJALVE 1983) (Fig. 1). The isocyanate component is able to either carbamoylate various cellular components or undergo intramolecular carbamoylation. While this type of reaction has received little investigative attention, as this review proceeds a potential role for carbamoylation of β cells in the etiology of SZ-induced diabetes will be suggested. The methyldiazohydroxide decomposes further to form a highly reactive carbonium ion, which is able to alkylate various cellular components such as DNA or protein or to react with H_2O to form methanol which can subsequently enter the 1-carbon pool. It is apparent that of these three potential sites for alkylation DNA would seem to be the most critical target since DNA alterations would have the most lasting effect

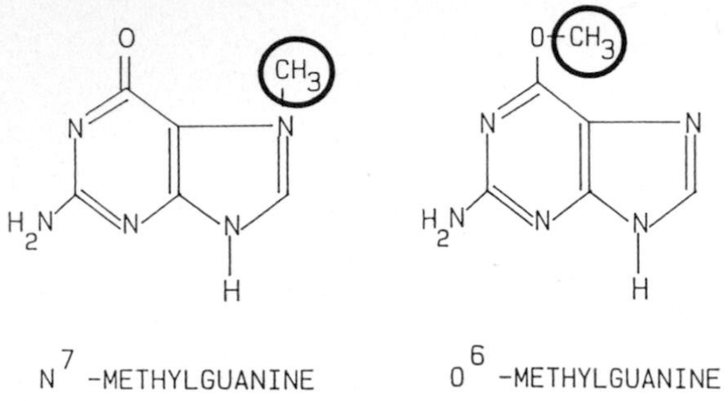

Fig. 2. Methylation of guanine at the N^7 and O^6 positions

on the organism. The carbonium ions formed by the decomposition of SZ are able to react with nucleophilic centers in DNA by a unimolecular (Sn1) reaction. These nucleophilic centers in DNA are the nitrogens and oxygens. The ring nitrogens are much stronger nucleophiles than the oxygens and, therefore, are alkylated more frequently. The predominant site for the alkylation of a ring nitrogen is at the 7 position of guanine [LEDOUX et al. 1986, Fig. 2]. Lesions in DNA of this type are removed by excision repair. Part of this excision repair process is the activation of the enzyme poly (ADP-ribose) synthetase to form poly (ADP-ribose) using NAD as a substrate [for a discussion of the role of poly (ADP-ribose) in excision repair see references (LEDOUX et al. 1986; WILSON et al. 1988)]. It has been hypothesized that in the β cell this enzyme becomes activated to such an extent that NAD becomes critically depleted, resulting in a cessation of cellular function and ultimately cell death (YAMAMOTO et al 1981). Although this hypothesis has been widely accepted, more recent studies have demonstrated that the toxic action of SZ is more complex than the overactivation of a single enzyme. LEDOUX et al. (1986) have shown that a cytotoxic concentration of SZ and an equimolar nonlethal concentration of its nitrosamide moiety methylnitrosourea alkylate the 7 position of guanine to the same extent and cause similar amounts of DNA strand breaks. Additional studies showed poly (ADP-ribose) synthetase also was activated to the same extent by equimolar concentrations of SZ and MNU. Although these studies exclude the possibility that SZ exerts its toxic effects solely by the critical depletion of nicotinamide adenine dinucleotide (NAD) due to the overactivation of poly (ADP-ribose) synthetase, the depletion of NAD as the final insult leading to cell death is not ruled out. Measurements of NAD concentrations in β cells following exposure to 1 m*M* SZ (toxic) or 1m*M* MNU (nontoxic) showed that NAD levels in MNU treated cells were 50% lower than control levels, while SZ-treated β cells had NAD concentrations that were only 13% of controls. Since SZ and MNU alkylated DNA to the same extent, caused comparable DNA strand breaks, and activated poly (ADP-ribose) synthetase in a similar fashion, it is probable that the depletion of NAD resulting from the activation of poly (ADP-ribose) synthetase would be that seen with MNU (approximately 50% of control). The drop in NAD concentration resulting from exposure to SZ (13%) must be due to other factors. Based on these findings, a new hypothesis to explain the lethal effects of a single high dose of SZ has been proposed (WILSON et al. 1988). It is speculated that on entering the β cell, SZ alkylates not only DNA, but key components necessary for the generation of ATP as well (e.g., glycolytic or mitochondrial enzymes). As part of the process to repair the DNA lesions, the enzyme poly(ADP-ribose) synthetase is activated with NAD as a substrate. The fall of NAD levels initiated by this process is not by itself lethal. However, when β cells are treated with SZ, concomitant with the activation of poly(ADP-ribose) synthetase is a drop in ATP formation most likely due to alkylation of vital enzymes. This fall in ATP generation would impair the resynthesis of NAD, causing the levels of this key cellular component to drop below critical levels. Therefore, it is speculated that it is the combination of two critical processes occurring simultaneously that allows a single bolus of SZ to selectively and rapidly destroy β cells.

Since SZ contains glucose in its structure, it is possible that the β cell may uniquely recognize and transport this toxin to some critical compartment that is peculiar to the β cell. Evidence that SZ does selectively alkylate key proteins in the β cell has been provided by recent studies using SZ labeled with ^{14}C at the 3′ carbon of the *N*-nitroso moiety. It was demonstrated that SZ is indeed sequestered differently in β cells than is the aglycone MNU. A greater proportion of carbonium ions alkylate β cell proteins following treatment with SZ than with treatment with MNU (WILSON et al. 1988). Although the proteins that specifically are alkylated have not yet been identified, it seems reasonable to propose that a significant proportion of them are related to the stimulus secretion mechanisms of the β cell. Several lines of evidence support this proposition. First, it is the glucose moiety in the structure of the SZ molecule that conveys its distinctive properties, since SZ and MNU are structurally identical except for glucose. Second, RINr cells, whose insulin release is not responsive to glucose stimulation, are insensitive to SZ toxicity (LEDOUX and WILSON 1988). They also appear to sequester MNU and SZ in a similar fashion, as evidenced by the fact that both chemicals alkylate the same proportion of DNA and protein (WILSON et al. 1988). Third, β cells treated in such a manner so that NAD levels drop to only 50% of controls will over time restore NAD concentrations to near normal values, but will still exhibit an insulin secretory defect in response to glucose stimulation (BOLAFFI et al. 1986). It should be mentioned that in this same study SZ also was found to suppress insulin secretion stimulated by phorbol ester in the absence of glucose. This finding indicates that some SZ induced damage to β cells occurs past the glucose recognition site and involves generalized postsignal events. Thus, even at sublethal concentrations, SZ causes a permanent defect in stimulated insulin secretion that is independent of NAD concentration. Therefore, the often cited Okamoto hypothesis for the overactivation of poly(ADP-ribose) synthetase is not only not valid for the critical events leading to cell death, it also fails to explain the alterations in cellular functions induced by SZ.

Since many key proteins associated with glucose transport and metabolism would be located at the cell membrane, methylation of certain of these proteins could alter their conformation and even cause them to be recognized as foreign by the immune system. The potential for lesions of this type to play a pathogenetic role in the multidose streptozotocin (MSZ) model of diabetes will be considered as this review proceeds.

While the N^7 position of guanine is the most frequently alkylated site in DNA, other targets also may be important. Carbonium ions formed by the decomposition of SZ are so highly reactive that they are able to react with unshared pairs of electrons in oxygen as well as nitrogen molecules. The most commonly alkylated base oxygen is at the O^6 position of guanine. This lesion is of potentially great interest. It has been correlated with toxicity in other systems (GOTH-GOLDSTEIN 1987) and may explain the progressive damage seen in cultured islets after a single exposure to SZ (BOLAFFI et al. 1986). This lesion may also play a role in the MSZ model of diabetes because methylation of this oxygen interferes with hydrogen bonding and allows guanine to mispair with thymine, thereby causing a point mutation (ZARBL et al. 1985; MATTES et al. 1988; DOLAN et al. 1988). A lesion of this type could cause the expression of a repressed gene that could code for a protein or other hapten not normally recognized by the immune system (e.g., a fetal protein or a retrovirus). In support of this notion is the finding that multiple low doses of SZ in CD-1 and C57BL/KsJ mice induce the expression of either C or A type retroviruses (APPEL et al. 1978). Additionally, it is conceivable that a mutation in a normally expressed gene would alter its product such that it would be rendered antigenic. In diabetes an example of a point mutation is found in individuals with type II diabetes who produce an aberrant insulin (HANEDA et al. 1983; SANZ et al. 1986). Direct evidence that *N*-nitroso compounds, like SZ, can produce this type of mutagenic alteration is provided by studies using *N'*-methyl-*N'* nitro-*N*-nitrosoguanidine. This chemical alkylates DNA and causes changes in both rat and human pepsinogen phenotypes (DEFIZE et al. 1988).

The repair of O^6 methyl guanine is different from that of the adducts formed in nitrogens. While adducts at the N^7 position of guanine or the N^3 position of adenine are removed by excision repair, methylation at the O^6 position of guanine is removed by a transfer protein. If this protein is present in low amounts or is not expressed in certain cells (e.g., β cells), then cell-specific mutagenesis could occur in the presence of a general exposure to a given toxin. This protein previously has been shown to be deficient in other tissues (DAY et al. 1980; SKLAR and SRAUSS 1980; SHILOH and BECKER 1981; HALL et al. 1985). However, to date, no studies have been reported evaluating this protein in the β cell.

Another target for alkylation of DNA, other than bases, is the phosphate backbone resulting in the formation of phosphotriesters (Fig 3). These lesions are formed by a variety of alkylating agents, including SZ, and have been reported to be slowly repaired or not repaired at all (SHOOTER and SLADE 1977; SHOOTER et al. 1977). Although the exact biological consequences of phosphotriesters have yet to be determined, it is established that these lesions cause conformational changes in DNA. These conformational changes could alter the binding of a repressor protein and lead to the expression of a normally silent gene whose product could elicit an immune reaction.

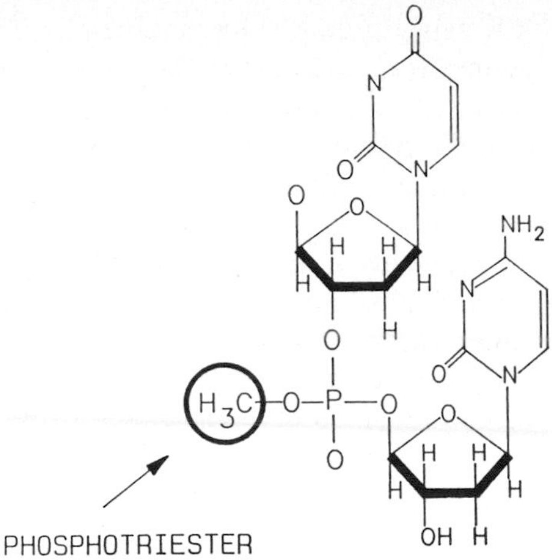

Fig. 3. Methylation of the phosphate backbone of DNA to form a phosphotriester

In summary, SZ could trigger diabetes by several mechanisms. First, its decomposition products can alter cellular membrane proteins so that they are no longer recognized as self. Alteration of proteins would include both alkylation and carbamoylation reactions. Second, SZ can alter DNA in such a manner that a previously silent gene is expressed or a normal protein is altered by point mutation. This could happen as a result of alkylation at the O^6 position of guanine which would allow this base to mispair with thymine or by alkylation of the phosphate backbone which would conformationally alter DNA.

3 The Multiple Low Dose Streptozotocin Model in Mice: Contributions of Immune System and Host Genotype

3.1 The Model

3.1.1 Description

An autoimmune etiology for IDDM in humans was initially suggested by the finding of insulitis in the islets of people with recent onset of IDDM (GEPTS 1965). This finding stimulated efforts to develop an animal model of diabetes in which insulitis was a prominent feature of the prediabetic and early diabetic pancreas. The multiple low dose streptozotocin (MSZ) induced diabetes model in male mice, developed by LIKE and ROSSINI (1976), provided researchers with one of the few experimental tools for analysis of the role of insulitis in β cell pathogenesis prior to the discovery of two spontaneously occurring rodent models, the BB rat and the NOD mouse. Outbred CD-1 males at 8 weeks of age were injected with 40 mg SZ per kg body weight (freshly prepared in citrate buffer, pH 4.2). These injections were administered once daily for 5 consecutive days (experiment days 1–5). Progressively severe glucose intolerance was noted at 7 days and by experiment day 31, a permanent, severe diabetic condition was produced. Heavy insulitis and disruption of islet cytoarchitecture was noted by experiment day 11. Preceding the arrival of the inflammatory cells was the induction in β cells of endogenous retroviruses, which were morphologically and immunocytochemically identified as type C (APPEL et al. 1978). Only males were susceptible; orchiectomy of CD-1 males blunted the level of MSZ-induced hyperglycemia, whereas testosterone treatment restored full sensitivity. Testosterone treatment of both ovariectomized and gonad-intact CD-1 females also increased hyperglycemic responsiveness to levels comparable with those observed in intact males (ROSSINI et al. 1978a).

3.1.2. Extrapolation of the Model to Inbred Strains

Since outbred CD-1 mice were not histocompatible and therefore not suitable for adoptive transfer studies, ROSSINI et al. (1977) compared MSZ susceptibility among males of various inbred mouse strains. Only C57BL/KsJ (BKs) exhibited the high sensitivity to MSZ induction of severe insulitis and hyperglycemia characteristic of CD-1 males. Interestingly, prenecrotic β cells in islets of MSZ-treated BKs males also showed induction of an endogenous β cell retroviral genome, that of an intracisternal type A particle [IAP (APPEL et al. 1978)]. The closely related C57BL/6J (B6) strain, as well as A/J, AKR/J, BALB/cJ, CBA/J, C3H/HeJ, and DBA/2J all exhibited various degrees of resistance to MSZ-induced insulitis and hyperglycemia when compared with highly susceptible BKs males (ROSSINI et al. 1977).

3.1.3 Sensitivity of Genetically Athymic Mice

IDDM etiopathogenesis is assumed to entail thymus dependent (auto) immunity against β cells, possibly mediated by cytotoxic T lymphocytes (CTL). Since CTL have been proposed as distal mediators of pathogenesis in MSZ-induced insulitis/diabetes (discussed in detail below), the question of whether genetically athymic (*nu*) mice are susceptible to MSZ-induced diabetes has been analyzed by at least six laboratories. One study showed "BALB/cBOM-*nu*/+" males to be susceptible and *nu*/*nu* males to be MSZ resistant unless reconstituted with T-lymphocyte enriched splenocytes from euthymic donors (PAIK et al. 1982a). Lethal irradiation eliminated sensitivity of *nu*/+ males, whereas sensitivity was restored by reconstitution of T-cell enriched splenocytes (PAIK et al. 1982a). This study unequivocally demonstrated the diabetogenic potential of T lymphocytes in this model, although the intensity of insulitis shown was very weak in comparison with insulitis seen in CD-1 or BKs islets following MSZ. However, this striking difference in susceptibility distinguishing euthymic from athymic mice has not been uniformly observed in other mouse colonies. In other studies involving "BALB/cBOM"-derived mice, euthymic mice were susceptible in two reports (BUSCHARD and RYGAARD 1978; NAKAMURA et al. 1984) and resistant (to 40 mg/kg × 5 days) in two other studies (KIESEL et al. 1981; BEATTIE et al. 1980). Similarly, "BALB/cBOM"-*nu/nu* males in various colonies have been shown to be partially resistant (BUSCHARD and RYGAARD 1978) or as sensitive as euthymic controls (NAKAMURA et al. 1984; BEATTIE et al. 1980). The basis for this controversy has recently been reviewed (LEITER 1985) and will be discussed briefly here.

Although many experimental variables can be enumerated to explain discordant findings [including variations in the diabetogenic potency of various batches of SZ, variations in the health status of the colonies, and in one instance, pooling data from males and females (BUSCHARD and RYGAARD 1978)], probably the most significant variable is the genetic heterogeneity among various BALB/c substrains. Whereas many biomedical researchers are fastidious about the quality of the chemicals they use in their research, they sometimes devote little consideration to the derivation and purity of their animals. The use of the strain symbol "BALB/c" to describe a mouse is equivalent to a diabetologist's use of the term "sugar" when glucose is actually the molecule being studied. There are numerous substrains of BALB/c mice, and the specification of the substrain is crucial because there is considerable variation in sensitivity to MSZ among certain well-characterized BALB/c substrains. The most problematic of these substrains are mice designated "BALB/cBOM"; these stocks represent incipient congenic strains produced in the course of transferring the *nu* mutation from the outbred NMRI background onto a BALB/c background. Quotation marks are used to denote not only nonstandard nomenclature, but also to denote a strain that appears incompletely inbred to a standard BALB/c background. For instance, in the studies described above showing absolute dependence of the model on T lymphocytes (PAIK et al. 1982a), mice at the fourth backcross to a BALB/c background were used, whereas in another study using mice after six backcrosses to BALB/c, both euthymic and athymic males were equally sensitive to MSZ-induced hyperglycemia, and thymus grafts into athymic mice did not further increase their responsiveness (NAKAMURA et al. 1984). Clearly, considerable genetic variability appears to differentiate the various *nu*- congenic stocks. Interpretation of "BALB/cBOM" studies has further been complicated by a report that the "BALB/cBOM" stock itself was genetically heterogeneous and thus should not be considered as an inbred BALB/c substrain (GUBBELS et al. 1985). The importance of the BALB/c background in determining the results obtained is best illustrated by comparing MSZ sensitivity of inbred BALB/cJ versus inbred BALB/cByJ males. Euthymic BALB/cJ males are strongly resistant to MSZ-induced hyperglycemia as originally reported by ROSSINI et al. (1977); however, euthymic males in the BALB/cByJ substrain were susceptible to MSZ-induced hyperglycemia, but in the absence of insulitis (LEITER 1985). Further aspects of genetic control of MSZ susceptibility in inbred BALB/c substrains will be discussed in depth in a later section.

The question of an obligatory requirement for thymus dependent immunity has also been tested in genetic backgrounds other than BALB/c. B6 males exhibit intermediate sensitivity to MSZ-induced hyperglycemia, with the diabetes syndrome developing in the absence of insulitis (LEITER 1982). Minimal inflammatory changes around the islets are characteristic of MSZ diabetogenesis on the B6 inbred background (ROSSINI et al. 1977; LEITER 1982). Since heavy insulitis was not associated with diabetogenesis in B6 mice, it was not surprising that C57BL/6JNIcrOu-*nu*/*nu* males were as susceptible to 40 mg/kg × 5 doses of SZ as euthymic littermate controls (LEITER 1982). On the other hand, since insulitis was a prominent characteristic of MSZ diabetogenesis in outbred CD-1 and inbred BKs euthymic males, it was unexpected that CD-1-*nu*/*nu* males and T-cell function-deficient BKs males were as susceptible as euthymic controls to the multiple dosage regimen employing 40 mg/kg × 5 (NAKAMURA et al. 1984; LEITER et al. 1983). Nevertheless, reduced sensitivity of CD-1-*nu*/*nu* males could be demonstrated at a lower dosage (30 mg/kg × 5); sensitivity could be enhanced by presence of a functional thymus graft, which in turn led to development of mild insulitis (NAKAMURA et al. 1984). The conclusion drawn in this latter study was that in strains where insulitis was a feature of MSZ pathogenesis, T-cell functions indeed contributed to MSZ sensitivity (NAKAMURA et al. 1984).

3.2 Pathogenetic Mechanisms of MSZ: Direct Cytotoxicity Versus Induction of Autoimmunity

3.2.1 Direct Cytotoxicity

Although each individual 40 mg/kg "subdiabetogenic" dose of SZ could not produce the same level of β cell necrosis and ensuing hyperglycemia as a single large diabetogenic dose (e.g., 160–200 mg/kg), the selective sensitivity of the β cell to this toxin would lead to the prediction that each "subdiabetogenic" dose was destroying significant numbers of *B* cells. If so, the cumulative effect of five such doses would be the erosion of pancreatic insulin reserves to levels allowing only marginal maintenance of glucose homeostasis. Indeed, exactly such a cumulative erosion of β cell mass and pancreatic insulin content has been demonstrated in BKs males prior to the development of peak insulitis (BONNEVIE-NIELSEN et al. 1981). Each subdiabetogenic dose of SZ destroyed or functionally impaired a percentage of the β cells, such that on experiment day 6 (1 day after the last MSZ injection), a 64% reduction in islet volume and an 84% reduction in insulin secretory capacity by perfused pancreas was shown (BONNEVIE-NIELSEN et al. 1981). Studies in vitro indicate that β cells surviving SZ-mediated lysis nevertheless remain functionally impaired (EIZIRIK et al. 1988). When islet insulin secretory capacity falls below 10%–15% of normal in BKs males mice, elevated plasma glucose levels reflect the pathophysiological process BONNEVIE-NIELSEN et al. 1981). The difficulty in analyzing the MSZ model, then, has been in separating what component of β cell loss and functional impairment was attributable to the direct β cell cytotoxicity of SZ versus secondary immunopathogenic damage mediated by lymphocytes in the insulitic infiltrates (if strong inflammation were present) or by macrophages (Mϕ) that precede lymphocytes into SZ-damaged islets (KOLB-BACHOFEN et al. 1988), independent of the presence or absence of insulitis.

3.2.2 Evidence for Autoimmune Pathogenesis

The combination of insulitis and endogenous retroviral gene expression elicited by MSZ treatment of CD-1 males clearly suggested that in addition to the recognized β-cytotoxic action of SZ, an immunopathologic response to β cell injury was also being elicited. In CD-1 males, injection of 0.22 mmol/mouse of either 3-O-methylglucose or nicotinamide immediately prior to each MSZ dose (to protect β cells from the direct cytotoxic effects of SZ) prevented hyperglycemia only for 2 weeks, after which time the animals became diabetic (ROSSINI et al. 1978b). Similarly, injections of anti-lymphocyte serum (ALS, 0.25 ml 3 times daily for 5 weeks) again retarded development of hyperglycemia during the course of the treatment, but diabetes developed shortly after treatment ceased. However, MSZ-treated CD-1 males given a combination of the 3-O-methylglucose and ALS treatments remained normoglycemic throughout the 14 week experimental period (ROSSINI et al. 1978b). These results supported the hypothesis that pathogenesis indeed required a cell-mediated immune response elicited by direct SZ-mediated β cell injury. Studies with athymic males reviewed above provided further evidence that thymic dependent immunity was capable of exacerbating MSZ-mediated damage. Although autoantibodies have been reported following subdiabetogenic doses of SZ (HUANG and TAYLOR 1981), male mice exhibiting B lymphocyte deficiency responded to MSZ-induced diabetogenesis. These data do not support a primary role for humoral immunity in this model (BLUE and SHIN 1984).

Since the germinal studies of Rossini and his colleagues, the pathogenic role of the immune system in the MSZ model has been extensively evaluated and a voluminous literature describing the effects of immunomodulatory compounds on the control of MSZ-induced hyperglycemia now exists. This literature, recently reviewed by KOLB (1987), shows that nearly all compounds or reagents suppressing T lymphocyte or macrophage function also partially suppress hyperglycemia development in MSZ-treated mice. These include antibodies against I-A, I-E, “I-J”, Thy-1, L3T4, Ly-2; irradiation; anti-inflammatory steroids; certain lectins; silica; and agents inhibiting serotonin enhanced vascular permeability [see KOLB 1987]. Only cyclosporin A failed to suppress diabetogenesis (KOLB et al. 1985), probably because it is also β cytotoxic in mice (ANDERSSON et al. 1984) and thus would compound MSZ-induced direct cytotoxicity to β cells. The literature, then, clearly establishes an immune system contribution to the erosion of β cell mass and resultant glucose intolerance. Indeed, β cell pathology induced in the MSZ model has occasionally been referred to as “autoimmune insulitis,” a term also employed to describe the pathogenesis of diabetes in the BB rat and the NOD mouse.

Is the pathogenesis induced by MSZ truly "autoimmune"? There are several features of diabetogenesis in BB rats and NOD mice which are not mimicked by the MSZ model. The autoimmune diabetes of BB rats and NOD mice is the consequence of genetically inherited immunoregulatory defects expressed at the level of bone marrow derived effector cells (SERREZE et al. 1988a; NAKANO et al. 1988). Leukocytes derived from bone marrow or spleen from NOD or BB donors can adoptively transfer diabetes to otherwise diabetes resistant radiation chimeras. Only one report has claimed a similar adoptive transfer of overt diabetes using splenocytes from MSZ-diabetic "BALB/cBOM" male donors (BUSCHARD and RYGAARD 1977). This study monitored the recipients for only a short term after injection and found the level of hyperglycemia (present already by 3 days posttransfer) was modest. Surprisingly, there was no requirement that the presumed effector cells be MHC matched with the recipient's "target" cells. As will be discussed below, "BALB/cBOM" mice appear to be noninbred. Successful adoptive transfer of a permanent diabetes using standard inbred mice has not been reported; possibly the transient rise in glucose in "BALB/cBOM" mice may have reflected a graft versus host response (FLOHR et al. 1983). More typical is the report of KIM and STEINBERG (1984) who failed to adoptively transfer diabetes into normal B6 males receiving splenocytes from MSZ-diabetic syngeneic donors. However, they were able to achieve a very mild and apparently transient rise in plasma glucose only if the recipients were first pretreated with a low dose of SZ prior to receiving splenocytes. Although transfers of splenocytes from MSZ-diabetic donors to naive recipients do not initiate a frank, permanent diabetes (chronic, severe hyperglycemia preceded by severe insulitis and accompanied by permanent insulinopenia), there has been a report of transfer of insulitis into "C57BL/6J/Bom"-*nu/nu* males (quotation marks are used to denote nonstandard nomenclature) without development of hyperglycemia (KIESEL et al. 1980). Given the problem of genetic heterogeneity in the "BALB/cBOM" stock that distinguish these mice from standard BALB/c substrains (GUBBELS et al. 1985), the "C57BL/6J/Bom" mouse may also prove not to be a standard B6 mouse. For example, MSZ treatment of C57BL/6J-*nu-nu* and nu/+ males at The Jackson Laboratory produced hyperglycemia in the absence of insulitis (LEITER 1982). Since the athymic mice were as sensitive to MSZ as the euthymic mice, it would not be expected that treatment with monoclonal antibodies against CD4 and CD8 T-lymphocyte subsets would be palliative. Yet when "C57BL/6J/Bom" males were treated with such monoclonals, the severity of hyperglycemia was significantly reduced (KANTWERK et al. 1987). This reduction of hyperglycemia was transitory since another laboratory reported hyperglycemia gradually developing after discontinuation of antibody treatments (DAYER-METROZ et al. 1988). A similar tautology exists for inbred BALB/cByJ males. Even though response of this strain to MSZ hyperglycemia occurs at The Jackson Laboratory in the absence of insulitis (LEITER 1985), treatment of BALB/cByJ males with anti-T lymphocyte monoclonal antibodies in another laboratory indeed attenuated hyperglycemia (HEROLD et al. 1987). The possibility that T-cell secretions may impair glucose tolerance whether or not insulitis is severe or minimal will be discussed in a later section.

Further evidence that MSZ-induced diabetes did not qualify as a model for spontaneously developing autoimmune diabetes has been provided by islet transplantation studies. Transplantation into MSZ-diabetic BKs recipients of syngeneic BKs islets in numbers sufficient to reverse hyperglycemia does not result in an autoimmune elimination of the engrafted islets at a time when insulitis is developing in the pancreatic islets (ANDERSSON 1979). This latter observation was seemingly inconsistent with the earlier study showing that ALS treatment blocked MSZ-induced hyperglycemia, but when treatment was discontinued, hyperglycemia rapidly ensued (ROSSINI et al. 1978b). If MSZ-induced diabetes were primarily autoimmune in etiology, then an immunological "memory" should have been engendered that would elicit rejection of syngeneic islet grafts, and the effector cells should be able to be concentrated and passively transferred. This apparent lack of immunological memory is explainable if it is assumed that the immune response is not autoimmune (i.e., a loss of tolerance to normal endogenous autoantigens has not occurred) as in the case of BB rats and NOD mice, but instead is specific for toxin modified β cells which would now be recognized as "non-self."

In the case where intact BKs islets transplanted into spleens of syngeneic male mice after the last injection of MSZ were not immunologically rejected, assuming that cell mediated immunity is a component of MSZ-mediated diabetogenesis, the best explanation as to why the transplanted islets were not rejected would be that they had not been modified by SZ. This implies that β cells, to stimulate immune recognition, must be altered by SZ to render them antigenically distinct from normal β cells (allo-recognition). Indeed, when BKs recipients of the intrasplenic BKs islet implants (that were functioning normally) were posttreated 3 or 6 weeks after islet transplantation with 25 mg/kg of SZ for 3 days, the transplanted islets could no longer maintain glucose homeostasis (SANDLER and ANDERSSON 1981). This "booster dose" phenomenon suggests that SZ alteration of β cells is required for immune recognition. This distinction separates the MSZ model from the BB rat and NOD mice, wherein autoreactive cells appear capable of eliminating islet grafts. Accordingly, MSZ-induced diabetes appears to represent a model for a distinct pathogenetic entity—diabetes elicited in a susceptible genotype by an extrinsic environmental toxin.

As described above, severe, permanent diabetes has not been convincingly transferred into normal recipients receiving syngeneic splenocytes from MSZ-treated males. Passive transfer of a modest hyperglycemia could only be achieved if the splenocyte recipient received at least one subdiabetogenic SZ dose (KIM and STEINBERG 1984). This would be logical if SZ induced a neoantigen either by derepression of a silent genome or by destroying enough β cells to release immunogenic quantities of an eclipsed antigen. In view of the findings of Klinkhammer et al. (1988) that T cells can distinguish between normal versus SZ-modified cells, MSZ treatments probably also alter the surfaces of surviving β cell by production of alkylated or carbamoylated structures. These in turn may be perceived as "non-self" by T cells, Mϕ, or NK cells. Alternatively, requirement for pretreatment of passive transfer recipients with subdiabetogenic dose(s) of SZ may affect the immune system components possibly by action against the suppressor limb of this system. Cytotoxicity produced by MSZ injections, like that produced by encephalomyocarditis (EMC) and Coxsackie virus infections, is not limited exclusively to β cells. SZ also injures many other organ systems and cell types, including immunohematopoietic stem cells (NICHOLS et al. 1981), as well as differentiated lymphocyte subclasses (ITOH et al. 1984) such that an immunosuppressive action is conceivable.

The MSZ model most resembles virus induced diabetes in mice, which is also male gender specific and regulated by testosterone (MORROW et al. 1980). Aspects of virus induced diabetes in mice have been reviewed (LEITER and WILSON 1988; YOON and RAY 1986). As in the case of MSZ, males of some, but not all inbred strains are susceptible to diabetes induced by EMC or Coxsackie virus. Thymic dependent immunity initially triggered against viral-infected β cells, but possibly extending to uninfected β cells or latently infected cells, possibly by molecular mimicry between a viral antigen and a β cell product, has been proposed as the mechanism of diabetes induction (BABU et al. 1985). Evidence both supporting and discounting this hypothesis exists (HAYNES et al. 1987; YOON et al. 1985).

3.2.3 Pathogenic Significance of Insulitis

The MSZ model has sometimes been described as "autoimmune insulitis." Indeed, some investigators are under the mistaken impression that there is no diabetes induction by MSZ unless there is precedent insulitis, and, similarly, if insulitis is detected, some assume that the inevitable consequence must be diabetes. Both of these conceptions are erroneous. At The Jackson Laboratory, a variety of inbred strains, in addition to those originally examined by ROSSINI et al. (1977), have been examined for sensitivity to MSZ-induced hyperglycemia and insulitis. Some, such as BALB/cByJ, C3H.SW/SnJ, C3H/OuJ, and C3HeB/FeJ, develop hyperglycemia without insulitis (LEITER 1985; SERREZE et al. 1988). On the other hand, diabetes resistant BKs females develop a pronounced insulitis following MSZ treatment, but do not exhibit overt hyperglycemia, presumably because of the protective effect of endogenous estrogens (PAIK et al. 1982b). The estrogen protection is probably not mediated via stimulation of immunoregulatory cells that suppress β cell specific CTL, but rather, following MSZ reduction of insulin concentrations to borderline levels of adequacy, may be associated with the known ability of estrogens to promote glucose homeostasis in the mouse (BAILEY and AHMED-SOROUR 1980). There are instances in which a very delayed onset development of MSZ-induced hyperglycemia is not preceded by an underlying insulitis. Strain C.B-17 male mice (derived from BALB/cAnIcr mice congenic for an Igh-1^b marker) exhibited moderate sensitivity to MSZ (E.H.L. laboratory, unpublished studies). As hyperglycemia was delayed in onset, mechanisms in addition to direct SZ cytotoxicity were assumed to exist. However, as with BALB/cByJ males, this hyperglycemia occurred in the absence of significant insulitis. The recessive mutation *scid* (severe combined immunodeficiency, Chr 16) occurred on this congenic background. C.B.-17-

scid/scid mice are characterized by failure to differentiate functional T and B lymphocytes, whereas all members of the myeloid series are present in normal numbers [Mφ, granulocytes NK cells, etc. (SHULTZ and SIDMAN 1987)]. The finding that C.B-17-*scid/scid* males also became hyperglycemic following MSZ treatment confirmed that there was not a requirement for lymphoid infiltration around the damaged islet. The interesting aspect of diabetogenesis in both normal and mutant genotypes was that in the absence of strong inflammatory responsiveness to the toxin administration, there was a significant reduction in the number of mice remaining severely hyperglycemic on experiment day 59. This suggests that when insulitis occurs, it is a localized expression of an inbred strain's level of inflammatory responsiveness to tissue injury. A strongly responding strain might not only develop insulitis as a localized response, but might also exhibit systemic changes [e.g., vascular lesions that enhance capillary permeabilities (BEPPU et al. 1987; SCHWAB et al. 1986)]. Accordingly, permanent diabetes would be effected in inbred strains with strong inflammatory responses (CD-1, BKs), whereas inbred strains responding with weak inflammatory responses (e.g., C.B-17-*scid/scid*) could preserve sufficient β cell viability to allow eventual regeneration of a minimally adequate insulin supply.

3.2.4 Cell Mediated Reactions Against β Cells

The assumption has been that cells cytotoxic to β cells are infiltrating into islets following MSZ treatment in strains in which insulitis is observed, even in inbred strains in which insulitis is slight. Infiltrating cells comprise Mφ as well as T and B lymphocytes; only *Mφ* and T lymphocytes have been implicated in pathogenesis (KOLB 1987). Mφ and neutrophils are probably the earliest infiltrating cells; pretreatment of mice with silica, a specific Mφ toxin, prevents severe hyperglycemia (OSCHILEWSKI et al. 1986). Insulin has been shown to be a Mφ chemoattractant (LEITER 1987), and Mφ will develop spontaneous cytotoxicity against islet cells in vitro (SCHWIZER et al. 1984). Two monokines, interleukin-1 (IL-1) and tumor necrosis factor (TNF), especially in combination with a T-cell cytokine, γ-interferon (γ-IFN), are extremely cytotoxic to cultured islet cells (NERUP et al. 1988). Splenocytes from MSZ-treated BKs mice have been shown to produce a modest chromium release from rat insulinoma cell targets (MCEVOY et al. 1984). The cell type(s) responsible for lysis have not been purified and were only transiently present; however, enrichment for T lymphocytes increased chromium release in this assay (MCEVOY et al. 1987). Evidence that β cell specific CTL are present in leukocytic infiltrates of MSZ-damaged islets is based on the immunocytochemical demonstration of both CD-4+ and CD-8+ T lymphocytes (HEROLD et al. 1987) as well as on the finding that monoclonal antibodies against L3T4 and Ly-2 (surface antigens marking these two lymphocyte subsets) block hyperglycemia induction (KANTWERK et al. 1987; HEROLD et al. 1987). Interestingly, one of these studies (HEROLD et al. 1987) utilized BALB/cByJ males, which show minimal leukocytic infiltration in comparison with CD-1 or BKs males (LEITER 1985). The implication is that systemic impairment of

T-lymphocyte function is therapeutic even in the absence of significant insulitis. Discussion of this possibility will be expanded in a later section.

3.2.5 Role of Cytokines in Modulation of MSZ-Induced Pathogenesis

Thymic dependent immune function is not always a prerequisite for MSZ diabetogenesis, even in BKs males where leukocytic infiltrates around SZ-damaged islets are heavy (LEITER et al. 1983). Mechanisms of β cell cytotoxicity involving cells of the immune system other than MHC-restricted CTLs have been suggested by recent studies implicating Mϕ in pathogenesis (KOLB-BACHOFEN et al. 1988; OSCHILEWSKI et al. 1986), as well as by studies in vitro showing that a variety of cytokines can compromise β cell function and viability (NERUP et al. 1988). IL-1, a Mϕ-secreted monokine, inhibits insulin secretion by mouse islet monolayers and is not cytotoxic by itself (OSCHILEWSKI et al. 1986), but it exerts strong β-cytolytic action in combination with γ-interferon, a lymphokine secreted by T cells (PUKEL et al. 1988). TNF, another monokine, also synergizes with γ-interferon to destroy β cells in vitro (PUKEL et al. 1988). Indeed, on the basis of these findings in vitro, NERUP et al. (1988) have proposed a pathogenetic model for IDDM involving local accumulation around β cells of toxic cytokines from Mϕ and activated T helper cells rather than "classical" MHC-restricted CTL. In addition to monokine secretion, activated Mϕ could be expected to secrete a variety of reactants toxic to β cells. That such cytokine interactions operate in the MSZ model is suggested by studies using CBA/Wehi mice. In vitro, it has not been possible to induce class II MHC (Ia) antigens on CBA islets cultured in the presence of γ-interferon alone (CAMPBELL et al. 1985). However, high concentrations of γ-interferon plus TNF act synergistically to induce Ia (CAMPBELL et al. 1985). In vivo, no Ia was found on CBA islet cells, but following five injections of 60 mg/kg SZ, Ia-positive cells around and in islets were observed by immunocytochemistry (FARR et al. 1988). Many of these cells at the islet periphery likely were infiltrating Ia-positive Mϕ, but some of the more interior cells likely were β cells induced to express Ia as a consequence of local increase in monokines and, possibly, lymphokines. The pathological consequences of MHC antigen expression on β cells remain controversial (FARR et al. 1988; FOULIS and BOTTAZZO 1988), but it is interesting that one of the indirect consequences of MSZ administration may be induction of MHC antigens on β cells. It is noteworthy that anti-inflammatory steroids such as hydrocortisone are strongly protective in the MSZ model (LEITER et al. 1983). Further, Mϕ would be expected to contribute to MSZ diabetogenesis under conditions in which circulating levels of insulin were limiting. Peripheral blood monocytes bind and degrade considerably more insulin than do lymphocytes, such that an increase in blood monocytes when insulin levels are barely adequate may contribute to overt hyperglycemia.

3.2.6 SZ Generation of β Cell "Neoantigens"

As already indicated, several strains of mice most susceptible to MSZ-induced hyperglycemia and insulitis (CD-1, BKs) also show induction of endogenous retroviral genes (type C or IAP). The IAP 73000 dalton structural core protein (p73) may serve as a model for a "neoantigen" in the sense that the purified protein is strongly immunogenic in mice, and antibody cross-reactivity studies indicate that p73 apparently shares an epitope (molecular mimicry) with both insulin and IgE binding factor (SERREZE et al. 1988b). IAP gene expression in murine β cells has been shown to be glucose inducible (LEITER et al. 1986). The glucose promotibility of these genes, coupled with their exclusive expression in β cells, but not α, δ, or PP cells, suggests that strains capable of retroviral expression must have a retroviral gene situated in the vicinity of the insulin I or II gene promoter region. If so, the SZ-induced retroviral expression in CD-1 and BKs β cells may reflect the response of β cell genomes to an increasingly hyperglycemic environment. There is immunoelectron microscopic evidence indicative of p73 transport to the β cell surface (LEITER and KUFF 1984), and expression of a β cell retrovirus has recently been associated with cyclophosphamide accelerated insulitis and diabetes development in NOD male mice (SUENAGA and YOON 1988). Cyclophosphamide, like SZ, can produce DNA damage. Thus, these agents may induce retroviral gene expression not only indirectly by effecting elevated plasma glucose concentrations, but perhaps also by acting directly at the DNA level. Inasmuch as Mϕ infiltration into the islets of MSZ-treated mice as well as NOD mice may be of pathogenic significance, it is likely that β cells induced to express endogenous retroviral neoantigens may attract Mϕ attention; and Mϕ infiltration, in turn, may not only damage surviving β cells (SCHWIZER et al. 1984), but may also serve as an antigen presenting cell and thus initiate increased leukocytic infiltration.

In addition to neoantigen presentation as a result of altered genetic expression, the ability of SZ to alter cell surface proteins suggests another mechanism whereby a neoantigen may be presented at the β cell surface. Following the protocol of KLINKHAMMER et al. (1988), popliteal lymph node T lymphocytes were isolated 12 days after priming BALB/cByJ females with a single injection of a subdiabetogenic quantity of SZ in complete Freund's adjuvant, and the primed T cells harvested were cocultured with BALB/cByJ islet cell monolayers pretreated with noncytotoxic levels of SZ or control medium alone (SERREZE et al. 1989). A specific T-lymphocyte blastogenic response was observed when the islet cells were SZ pretreated, but control islet cultures did not serve as stimulators, suggesting that β cell surface proteins altered by SZ may indeed be immunogenic (SERREZE et al. 1989).

3.3 Genetic Control of Susceptibility to MSZ

3.3.1 Role of Major Histocompatibility Complex

In humans, BB rats, and NOD mice, an important susceptibility locus for IDDM has been linked to the major histocompatibility complex (MHC). In the mouse, the *H-2* complex on chromosome 17 contains important immunoregulatory loci.

Initially, studies employing *H-2* congenic stocks of mice on the C57BL/10J (B10) inbred background indicated no association of the *H-2^b^* haplotype with MSZ sensitivity (KROMANN et al. 1982), but subsequent analyses using various congenic stocks did suggest a gene controlling sensitivity mapped proximal to the *H-2^d^* locus, with *H-2^b^* haplotypes usually associated with resistant phenotypes (KIESEL et al. 1983). However, the MHC associations were not consistent when different inbred strain background were analyzed, indicating the MSZ sensitivity must be controlled by at least one non-MHC gene (KIESEL et al. 1983; WOLF et al. 1984; LE et al. 1985). For example, although the *H-2^b^* haplotype on B10 and BALB/c backgrounds appeared protective (KIESEL et al. 1983; WOLF et al. 1984), the same haplotype in C3H.SW/SnJ was not (LE et al. 1985). Indeed, analysis of susceptibility within C3H substrains indicated that non-MHC genes determining sensitivity to endogenous androgens were the primary modifiers of susceptibility to MSZ-induced hyperglycemia (LE et al. 1985). An androgen sensitive retroviral enhancer element regulating class III MHC gene expression (sex limited protein, *Slp*) in males has recently been found proximal to the *H-2^d^* locus (STAVEHAGEN and ROBINS 1988). Thus, strain and gender specific control of tissue androgen/estrogen balance could regulate MHC gene expression at a secondary level. A critical evaluation of the potential protective role of the *H-2^b^* haplotype was performed by transferring it from the relatively MSZ- and insulitis-resistant B6 background onto the highly susceptible BKs background. No loss of sensitivity to insulitis and hyperglycemia induction was observed in BKs.B6-*H-2^b^* congenic males at the 7th backcross generation (LEITER et al. 1987). Thus, this lack of a strong MHC association in the MSZ model is in contrast to IDDM in humans, BB rats, and NOD mice, but is consistent with the models of virally induced diabetes in male mice (YOON et al. 1985). In both the viral and MSZ models, increased sensitivity to or availability of endogenous androgens appears to be a common feature of male mice from those inbred strains showing high sensitivity to hyperglycemia induction (LEITER et al. 1987).

The most intensive effort to map a genetic locus controlling responsiveness to MSZ has been conducted in two closely related BALB/c substrains, the resistant BALB/cJ and the susceptible BALB/cByJ strain. These two substrains differ at very few typed genetic loci; they share *H-2^d^* haplotype but differ in expression of the linked *Qa-2* gene. In (BALB/cByJ × BALB/cJ) outcross, F1 hybrid were MSZ resistant, indicating BALB/cByJ male susceptibility was recessive. Backcross of the resistant F1 hybrids to the susceptible BALB/cByJ parental strain produced 1:1 segregation of susceptible versus resistant phenotypes, indicating that a single locus was segregating (LEITER et al. 1989). No linkage to polymorphic markers on Chr 17 or Chr 5 was found; again, genes regulating sensitivity to endogenous androgen rather than MHC genes appeared to be a major determinant. A report showing enhanced female susceptibility to SZ following phenobarbital treatment suggested that genetic differences in cytochrome P450 activation following SZ treatment may underlie differential inbred strain, as well as gender dimorphic sensitivities (MACLAREN et al. 1980). However, SZ is a nitrosamide, rather than a nitrosamine, and does not require metabolism by cytochrome P450 for its decomposition to reactive species. Therefore, it is highly improbably that the cytochrome P450 system could contribute to the toxic effects of SZ. A more likely explanation would be that other effects of phenobarbital on the β cell (e.g., inhibition of alkyltransferase) account for the enhancing effect of this chemical on the toxic action of SZ. Although cytochrome P450 enzymes may not be directly related to the toxic effects of SZ, it is possible that the genes controlling these enzymes may be linked to genes associated with susceptibility and resistance. This possibility currently is under investigation in the BALB/c substrains described above.

A previous study had concluded that suppressor cells controlled MSZ resistance of "BALB/cBom" males since immunomodulation by a relatively low dose of cyclophosphamide (70 mg/kg body weight) enhanced hyperglycemic responsiveness (KIESEL et al. 1981). Interestingly, a difference was found between the BALB/cJ and BALB/cByJ substrains in their ability to activate T-lymphocyte suppressor-inducer function in a syngeneic mixed lymphocyte reaction [SMLR (SERREZE et al. 1989)]. The SMLR represents a T cell response in vitro to self-MHC class II; a portion of the responding cells (SMLR blasts) have been demonstrated to induce suppression of syngeneic T-lymphocyte responses, including those to alloantigens in a mixed lymphocyte reaction (MLR). T lymphocytes from both BALB/cJ and BALB/cByJ mice demonstrate strong blastogenic responses in a SMLR. SMLR blasts generated using responder T cells from BALB/cJ spleens indeed suppressed the response of BALB/cJ T lymphocytes in a MLR. In contrast, SMLR-generated BALB/cByJ T lymphocytes activated in a SMLR failed to suppress BALB/cByJ responses in an MLR (SERREZE et al. 1989). Genetic analysis of this BALB/cByJ defect in suppressor-inducer cell function showed that the trait was inherited in the same recessive manner as BALB/cByJ susceptibility to MSZ. That is, in (BALB/cJ, × BALB/cByJ)F1 hybrids, the suppressor dysfunction was recessive, and upon backcross to the suppression defective BALB/cByJ parental strain, a 1:1 segregation of the trait was observed (SERREZE et al. 1989). Since the BALB/cByJ trait for MSZ susceptibility segregated in an identical fashion, it is tempting to infer that the recessive defect in BALB/cByJ T suppressor function is identical to the recessive trait controlling MSZ sensitivity of this substrain. However, in the absence of a polymorphic genetic marker demonstrating that the locus controlling both of these physiological responses (hyperglycemia, deficient suppression) is on the same chromosome, the relation between the two responses can not be resolved. Although it might seem logical to test backcross mice susceptible to MSZ-induced diabetes for concordance with the SMLR function deficiency, such an analysis has not been done because comparisons of immunological functions between diabetic versus non-diabetic groups of mice would be confounded by the combined suppressive effects of SZ and diabetes on immune function (ITOH et al. 1984). An observation favoring the hypothesis that a deficiency in T-cell function and diabetes susceptibility are related is that BALB/cByJ males are also susceptible to EMC virus-induced hyperglycemia, which is also modulatd by T-lymphocyte functions (HAYNES et al. 1987). Assuming that defective suppression of certain T-lymphocyte functions may contribute to hyperglycemia development, it does not necessarily follow that this contribution must be via CTL activation and insulitis development. It should be recalled that insulitis is not a feature of MSZ-induced diabetogenesis in BALB/cByJ males (LEITER 1985). Although the T suppressor function defect could underlie diabetogenic sensitivity in both the virus and the MSZ models, the basis for the susceptibility may be increased systemic T lymphocyte activities, including secretion of neuroendocrinelike peptides modulating glucose homeostasis. This possibility will be discussed in detail below.

3.4 Interrelationships Between the Immune System and the Neuroendocrine System: A New Hypothesis for Explaining Immune System Interaction in the MSZ Model

3.4.1 The Neuroimmunoendocrine Axis and Diabetes

In the discussion of MSZ pathogenesis up to this point, only two narrow parameters have been considered: (1) direct β-cytotoxic action of SZ and (2) secondary stimulation of cell mediated autoimmunity against damaged β cells. This narrow focus accurately reflects the literature; the model has heretofore always been viewed solely on the basis of how the toxin and the immune system interact with β cells. A clearer understanding of this model is achieved by a broader view of how glucose homeostasis is maintained in a mouse. Other neuroendocrine organs, including the hypothalamus, pituitary, adrenals, gonads, as well as muscle and liver all play essential roles. Indeed, the diabetogenic role of androgens and palliative role of estrogens were recognized at the inception of the model, but scant investigation into the biochemical basis for this gonadal dependency, or for relationship between MSZ sensitivity and secretions from other organ systems, has been performed.

A recent symposium volume enumerates the accumulating evidence for bidirectional communication between the immune system and neuroendocrine organs (JANKOVIC et al. 1987). That a neuroimmunoendocrine axis is important in the MSZ model is illustrated by the report that caging stress (as measured by elevated plasma corticosterone level) accelerated hyperglycemic induction in BKs males (MAZELIS et al. 1987). Although it might be assumed that the mechanism entailed corticosterone induced thymolytic or other immunosuppressive effects (inhibition of suppressor cells?), the rapidity of the hyperglycemic induction in this study suggested that adrenal glucocorticoids were directly acting to elevate plasma glucose. Glucose output from liver and muscle tissue during interprandial periods represents a major component of plasma glucose; glucocorticoids, in concert with glucagon and epinephrine, are important regulators of gluconeogenesis and glucose release from these tissues. The hypothalamus, via secretion of corticotropin releasing factor (CRF), stimulates

ACTH release from the anterior pituitary, which in turn, stimulates adrenal output of glucocorticoids. Cells of the immune system apparently enter into this neuroendocrine regulatory circuit in several ways.

3.4.2 Lymphoid-Adrenal Axis

A surprising finding has been that activation of the immune system by certain antigens, especially viral antigens, can result in release of bioactive ACTH and growth hormone (GH) from lymphoid cells (Harbour and Blalock 1987). The entire proopiomelanocortin (POMC) gene is apparently transcribed in these cells, leading to production of β endorphin as well as ACTH (Harbour and Blalock 1987). Another lymphocyte product, glucocorticoid increasing factor (GIF) has been described in rats (Besedovsky et al. 1985). The lymphocyte derived ACTH would be anticipated to synergize with ACTH of pituitary origin in stimulating corticosteroid secretion and thereby antagonizing the antihyperglycemic action of limited quantities of insulin following MSZ erosion of the β cell mass. POMC gene products, in turn, affect the function of lymphoid cells (Morley et al. 1987). The depressed suppressor function of BALB/cByJ could reflect underlying endocrinological differences. Indeed, neuroendocrine differences between the diabetes resistant BALB/cJ males diabetes susceptible males from other BALB/c substrains are well established. Of all BALB/c substrains, only BALB/cJ males exhibit strong fighting behavior; this behavioral difference, controlled by a single gene, was associated with a twofold increased activity of three adrenal medullary catecholamine biosynthetic enzymes in BALB/cJ (Ciaranello et al. 1974). The point is that the "stressability" of the inbred strain background must be considered when hyperglycemia is the end point. Probably the most controversial report to date in the field of the immunology of diabetes has been that claiming passive transfer of diabetes into *nu/nu* mice by leukocytes from IDDM patients (Buschard et al. 1978). When the study was repeated with appropriate controls, glycemic changes and changes in islet structure were concluded to reflect "nonspecific stress reaction" rather than adoptive transfer of an autoimmune disease (Uehara et al. 1987). Because the mouse is such a conveniently utilized research tool, the biology of this living organism is sometimes overlooked in the rush to establish "immunological truths." Future claims of disease transfer from man to mouse should be accepted only if a rigorous battery of controls (for stress, possibly mediated in part via leukocyte secretions) are provided.

3.4.3 IL-1 and Glucose Homeostasis

The evidence that cells of the reticuloendothelial system, especially Mϕ, play an important role in maintenance of glucose homeostasis has already been discussed, as has the potential pathogenic significance of Mϕ IL-1 secretion directly into the environment of SZ-damaged β cells. IL-1 can also affect glucose homeostatic mechanisms indirectly by affecting the hypothalamus (Uehara et al. 1987), by stimulating CRF release which in turn stimulates ACTH release, or possibly by stimulating pituitary ACTH release directly (BESEDOVSKY et al. 1986). Obviously, IL-1, by stimulating T-lymphocyte activation, could also stimulate ACTH release from lymphoid tissues (HARBOUR and BLALOCK 1987). IL-1, therefore, could modulate plasma glucose levels indirectly by stimulating ACTH release from lymphocytes. However, chronic treatment of mice with exogenous IL-1 actually suppressed key enzymes of hepatic gluconeogenesis (HILL et al. 1986), such that it is unclear whether increases in blood levels of ACTH and, secondarily, of glucocorticoids elicited by IL-1 would necessarily produce elevated plasma glucose.

If leukocyte secretions can contribute to glucose intolerance, the expectation would be that mice whose immune systems had been stimulated by challenge with environmental viruses would respond to MSZ more strongly than would mice whose immune systems had not been recently challenged. In the MSZ model, exposure to environmental viruses apparently had this effect; i.e., the more stimulated the immune system, the stronger the hyperglycemic responsiveness of the male mice to MSZ. This was illustrated by two separate colonies of BALB/cByJ mice studied at The Jackson Laboratory (LEITER et al. 1989). Males from the original colony studied exhibited a strong hyperglycemic responsiveness by experiment day 24; this responsiveness was associated with serological evidence of an enzootic infection by pneumonia virus of mice [PVM; (LEITER et al. 1989)] When the colony was rederived to eliminate completely any PVM carriers, the male responsiveness to MSZ, while still present, was attenuated such that peak hyperglycemia, formerly seen by experiment day 24, was now observed at experiment day 52 (LEITER et al. 1989). Thus, the specific pathogen free status of a colony may be one of the variables controlling MSZ sensitivity, with secretions from leukocytes from mice having more "robust" immune systems impairing glycemic control by synergizing with the cumulative diabetogenic effects of each SZ dose. It is noteworthy in this regard that mice or rats pretreated with complete Freund's adjuvant (an immunostimulant) exhibited heightened sensitivity to diabetes induction by MSZ (MCEVOY et al. 1987; ZIEGLER et al. 1984, 1988). This exacerbation of hyperglycemia by immunostimulation in the MSZ model contrasts with the autoimmune diabetes prone NOD males in which precisely the inverse response has been demonstrated. In Japan, NOD males reared under germ free conditions develop a much higher diabetes incidence than those in conventional colonies (SUZUKI et al. 1987). Experimental virus infections of NOD mice actually suppress the development of overt diabetes (OLDSTONE 1988), probably by stimulating immunoregulatory (suppressor?) networks.

4 Summary and Conclusions

The MSZ diabetic male mouse represents one of the most useful tools available to researchers interested in analyzing the consequences of insulin dependent diabetes in male mice. In contrast to the high mortality induced by single high doses of SZ, protracted administration of smaller SZ dosages yields a more stable diabetic condition. Moreover, in insulitis prone strains such as BKs, the model allows "synchronization" of β cell destruction such that the inflammatory events occur on a predictable timescale. The MSZ-diabetic mouse represents a diabetic condition in which the primary etiopathologic effect is produced by an environmental toxin, and not by a genetically programmed loss of tolerance to β cell specific antigens. In this regard, etiopathogenesis in the MSZ model is quite distinct from that underlying autoimmune type I diabetes in humans, NOD mice, and BB rats, and it is probably not appropriate to refer to pathogenesis in the MSZ model as one of "autoimmune insulitis" as has sometimes been done. The fact that insulitis in the MSZ model may not be "autoimmune," but may actually be a normal response to either tissue damage or to β cells that have been structurally modified by a chemical, makes the model of special interest. Clearly, there is no single cause of insulin dependent diabetes, with disease induction representing a genetic susceptibility interacting with environmental triggers, such as toxins in the diet (including nitrosamines and fungal metabolites) as well as pathogenic viruses. The MSZ model will continue to be actively investigated because of insights it will afford regarding the genetic bases for susceptibility and resistance to diabetogenic environmental toxins. The model will be of further value by contributing to knowledge of the complicated interactions between pancreatic islet cells, other endocrine cells, and leukocytes in maintenance of glucose homeostasis.

References

Ames BN (1983) Dietary carcinogens and anticarcinogens: oxygen radicals and degenerative diseases. Science 221: 1256–1264

Andersson A (1979) Islet implantation normalizes hyperglycemia caused by streptozotocin-induced insulitis. Lancet 1: 581–584

Andersson A, Borg H, Hallberg A, Hellerstrom C, Sandler S, Schnell A (1984) Long-term effects of cyclosporin A on cultured mouse pancreatic islets. Diabetologia 27: 66–69

Appel MC, Rossini AA, Williams RM, Like AA (1978) Viral studies in streptozotocin-induced pancreatic insulitis. Diabetologia 15: 327–336

Babu PG, Huber SA, Craighead JE (1985) Immunology of viral diabetes. Surv Synth Pathol Res 4: 1–7

Beattie G, Lannom R, Lipsick J, Kaplan NO, Osler AG (1980) Streptozotocin-induced diabetes in athymic and conventional BALB/c mice. Diabetes 29: 146–150

Bailey CJ, Ahmed-Sorour H (1980) Role of ovarian hormones in the long term control of glucose homeostasis. Effects on insulin secretion. Diabetologia 19: 475–481

Beppu H, Maruta K, Kurner T, Kolb H (1987) Diabetogenic action of streptozotocin: essential role of membrane permeability. Acta Endocrinol 114: 90–95

Besedovsky HO, Del Rey A, Sorkin E, Lotz W, Schwulera U (1985) Lymphoid cells produce an immunoregulatory glucocorticoid increasing factor (GIF) acting through the pituitary gland. Clin Exp Immunol 59: 622–628

Besedovsky H, Del Rey A, Sorkin E, Dinarello A (1986) Immunoregulatory feedback between IL-1 and glucocorticoid hormones. Science 233: 652–654

Blue ML, Shin SI (1984) Diabetes induction by subdiabetogenic doses of streptozotocin in

BALB/cBOM mice. Noninvolvement of host B-lymphocyte functions. Diabetes 33: 105–110
Bolaffi JL, Nowlan RE, Cruz L, Grodsky GM (1986) Progressive damage of cultured pancreatic islets after single early exposure to streptozotocin. Diabetes 35: 1027–1033
Bolaffi JL, Nagamatsu S, Harris J, Grodsky GM (1987) Protection by thymidine, an inhibitor of polyadenosine diphosphate ribosylation, of streptozotocin inhibition of insulin secretion. Endocrinology 120: 2117–2122
Bonnevie-Nielsen V, Steffes MW, Lernmark A (1981) A major loss in islet mass and B-cell function precedes hyperglycemia in mice given multiple low doses of streptozotocin. Diabetes 30: 424–429
Brosky G, Logothetopoulos J (1969) Streptozotocin diabetes in the mouse and guinea pig. Diabetes 18: 606–613
Buschard K, Rygaard J (1977) Passive transfer of streptozotocin induced diabetes mellitus with spleen cells. Acta Pathol Microbiol Immunol Scand [C] 85: 469–472
Buschard K, Rygaard J (1978) Is the diabetogenic effect of streptozotocin in part thymus-dependent? Acta Pathol Microbiol Immunol Scand [C] 86: 23–27
Buschard K, Madsbad S, Rygaard J (1978) Passive transfer of diabetes mellitus from man to mouse. Lancet 2: 908–910
Campbell IL, Wong GHW, Schrader JW, Harrison LC (1985) Interferon-gamma enhances the expression of the major histocompatibility class I antigens on mouse pancreatic β cells. Diabetes 34: 1205–1209
Campbell IL, Oxbrow L, Koulmanda M, Harrison LC (1988) IFN-gamma induces islet cell MHC antigens and inhances autoimmune, streptozotocin-induced diabetes in the mouse. J Immunol 140: 1111–1116
Ciaranello RD, Lipsky A, Axelrod J (1974) Association between fighting behavior and catecholamine biosynthetic enzyme activity in two inbred mouse sublines. Proc Natl Acad Sci USA 71: 3006–3008
Cooperstein SJ, Watkins D (1981) Action of toxic drugs on islets. In: Cooperstein SJ, Watkins D (eds) The islets of Langerhans. Academic, New York, pp 387–425
Craighead JE (1978) Current views of insulin -dependent diabetes mellitus. N Engl J Med 299: 1439–1445
Day RS, Ziolkowski CHJ, Scudiero DA, Meyer SA, Lubiniecki AS, Girardi AJ, Galloway SM, Bynum GD (1980) Defective repair of alkylated DNA by human tumour SV40 transformed human cell strains. Nature 288: 724–727
Dayer-Metroz MD, Kimoto M, Izui S, Vassalli P, Renold AE (1988) Effect of helper and/or cytotoxic T-lymphocyte depletion on low-dose streptozotocin-induced diabetes in C57BL/6J mice. Diabetes 37: 1082–1089
Defize J, Derodra JK, Riddell RH, Hunt RH (1988) Changes in rat and human pepsinogen phenotypes induced by *N'*-methyl-*N'*nitro-*N*-nitrosoguanidine. Cancer 62: 1958–1961
Dolan ME, Oplinger M, Pegg AE (1988) Sequence specificity of guanine alkylation and repair. Carcinogenesis 9: 2139–2143
Dulin WE, Soret MG (1977) Chemically and hormonally induced diabetes. In: Volk BW, Wellman KF (eds) The diabetic pancreas. Planum, New York, pp 425–466
Eisenbarth GS (1986) Type I diabetes mellitus: a chronic autoimmune disease. N Engl J Med 314: 1360–1368
Eizirik Dl, Sandler S, Welsh N, Hellerstrom C (1988) Preferential reduction of insulin production in mouse pancreatic islets maintained in culture after streptozotocin exposure. Endocrinology 122: 1242–1249
Farr AG, Mannschreck JW, Anderson SK (1988) Expression of class II MHC antigens in murine pancreas after streptozotocin-induced insulitis. Diabetes 37: 1373–1379
Flohr K, Kiesel U, Freytag G, Kolb H (1983) Insulitis as a consequence of immune dysregulation: further evidence. Clin Exp Immunol 53: 605–613
Foulis AK, Bottazzo GF (1988) Insulitis in the human pancreas. In: Lefebvre PJ, Pipeleers DG (eds) The pathology of the endocrine pancreas in diabetes. Springer, Berlin Heidelberg New York, pp 41–52
Gepts W (1965) Pathological anatomy of the pancreas in juvenile diabetes mellitus. Diabetes 14: 619–633
Goth-Goldstein R (1987) MNNG-induced partial phenotypic reversion of Mer- cells. Carcinogenesis 8: 1449–1453
Gubbels E, Poort-Keesom R, Hilgers J (1985) Genetically contaminated BALB/c nude mice. Curr Top Microbiol Immunol 122: 86–88

Hall J, Bresil H, Montesano R (1985) O^6-Alkyguanine DNA alyltransferase activity in monkey, human and rat liver. Carcinogenesis 6: 209–211

Haneda M, Chan SJ, Kwok SCM, Rubenstein AH, Steiner DF (1983) Studies on mutant human insulin genes: identification and sequence analysis of a gene encoding [Ser^{S24}] insulin. Proc Natl Acad Sci USA 80: 6366–6370

Harbour DV, Blalock JE (1987) Leukocyte production of endorphins. In: Jankovic DB, Markovic BM, Spector NH (eds) Neuroendocrine interactions: proceedings of the second international workshop on neuroimmunomodulation. Ann NY Acad Sci 496: 192–195

Hawksworth GM, Hill JJ (1974) The in vivo formation of N-nitrosamines in the rabbit bladder and their subsequent absorption. Br J Cancer 29: 353–358

Haynes MK, Huber SA, Craighead JE (1987) Helper-inducer T-lymphocytes mediate diabetes in EMC-infected BALB/cByJ mice. Diabetes 36: 877–881

Hedler L, Marquardt P (1968) Occurrence of diethylnitrosamine in some samples of food. Food Cosmet Toxicol 6: 341–349

Helgason T, Jonasson MR (1981) Evidence for a food additive as a cause of ketosis-prone diabetes. Lancet 2: 716–720

Helgason T, Even SWB, Ross IS, Stowers JM (1982) Diabetes produced in mice by smoked cured mutton. Lancet 2: 1017–1021

Herold KC, Montag AG, Fitch FW (1987) Treatment with anti-T-lymphocyte antibodies prevents induction of insulitis in mice given multiple doses of streptozotocin. Diabetes 36: 796–801

Hill MR, Stith ED, McCallum RE (1986) Interleukin 1: a regulatory role in glucocorticoid-regulated hepatic metabolism. J Immunol 137: 858–862

Huang SW, Taylor GE (1981) Immune insulitis and antibodies to nucleic acids induced with streptozotocin in mice. Clin Exp Immunol 43: 425–429

Itoh M, Junauchi M, Sato K, Kisamori S, Fukuma N, Hirooka Y, Nihei N (1984) Abnormal lymphocyte function precedes hyperglycemia in mice treated with multiple low doses of streptozotocin. Diabetologia 27: 109–112

Jankovic DB, Markovic BM, Spector NH (1987) Neuroendocrine interactions: proceedings of the second international workshop on neuroimmunomodulation. Ann NY Acad Sci 496: 756–764

Kantwerk G, Cobbold S, Waldmann H, Kolb H (1987) L3T4 and Lyt-2 T cells are both involved in the generation of low-dose streptozotocin-induced diabetes in mice. Clin Exp Immunol 70: 585–592

Karam JH, Lewitt P, Young C, Nowlain R, Frankel B, Fujiya H, Freedman Z, Grodsky G (1980) Insulinopenic diabetes after rodenticide (Vacor) ingestion: a unique model of acquired diabetes in man. Diabetes 29: 971–978

Kiesel U, Freytag G, Kolb H (1980) Transfer of experimental autoimmune insulitis by spleen cells in mice. Diabetologia 19: 516–520

Kiesel U, Greulich B, Moume CMS, Kolb H (1981) Induction of experimental autoimmune diabetes by low dose streptozotocin treatment in genetically resistant mice. Immunol Lett 3: 227–230

Kiesel U, Falkenberg FW, Kolb H (1983) Genetic control of low-dose streptozotocin-induced autoimmune diabetes in mice. J Immunol 130: 1719–1722

Kim YT, Steinberg C (1984) Immunologic studies on the induction of diabetes in experimental animals. Cellular basis for the induction of diabetes by streptozotocin. Diabetes 33: 771–777

Klinkhammer C, Popowa P, Gleichmann H (1988) Specific immunity to the diabetogen streptozotocin: cellular requirements for induction of lymphoproliferation. Diabetes 37: 74–80

Kneip TJ, Daisey JM, Solomon JJ, Hershmann RJ (1983) *N*-nitroso compounds: evidence for their presence in airborne particles. Science 221: 1045–1046

Kolb H (1987) Mouse models of insulin dependent diabetes: low-dose streptozotocin-induced diabetes and nonobese diabetic (NOD) mice. Diabetes Metab Rev 3: 751–778

Kolb H, Oschilewski M, Schwab E, Oschilewski U, Kiesel U (1985) Effect of cycloporin A on low-dose streptozotocin diabetes in mice. Diabetes Res 2: 191–193

Kolb-Bachofen V, Epstein S, Kiesel U, Kolb H (1988) Low dose streptozotocin-induced diabetes in mice. Electron microscopy reveals single cell insulitis before diabetes onset. Diabetes 37: 21–27

Kromann H, Christy M, Egeberg J, Lernmark A, Nerup J (1982) Absence of H-2 genetic influence on streptozotocin-induced diabetes in mice. Diabetologia 23: 114–118

Krowlewski A, Warram JH, Rand LI, Kahn CR (1987) Epidemiological approach to the etiology of type I diabetes mellitus and its complications. N Engl J Med 317: 1390–1398

Lazarus IS, Sharpiro IH (1973) Influence of nicotinamde and pyridine nucleotides on streptozotocin and alloxan-induced pancreatic B-cell cytotoxicity. Diabetes 22: 499–506

Le PH, Leiter EH, Leyendecker JR (1985) Genetic control of susceptibility to streptozotocin diabetes in inbred mice: effect of testosterone and H-2 haplotype. Endocrinology 116: 2450–2455

LeDoux SP, Wilson GL (1984) Effects of streptozotocin on a clonal isolate of rat insulinoma cells. Biochim Biochim Biophys Acta 804: 387–392

LeDoux SP, Woodley SE, Patton NJ, Wilson GL (1986) Mechanisms of nitrosoamide-induced β cell damage: alterations in DNA. Diabetes 35: 866–872

Lefebvre PJ (1988) Clinical forms of diabetes mellitus. In: Lefebvre PJ, Pipeleers DG (eds) The pathology of the endocrine pancreas in diabetes, Springer, Berlin Heidelberg New York, pp 1–16

Leiter EH (1982) Multiple low dose streptozotocin-induced hyperglycemia and insulitis in C57BL mice: influence of inbred background, sex, and thymus. Proc Soc Natl Acad Sci USA 79: 630–634

Leiter EH (1985) Differential susceptibility of BALB/c sublines to diabetes induction by multi-dose streptozotocin treatment. Curr Top Microbiol Immunol 122: 78–85

Leiter EH (1987) Murine macrophages and pancreatic β cells. Chemotactic properties of insulin and β-cytostatic action of interleukin 1. J Exp Med 166: 1174–1179

Leiter EH, Kuff EL (1984) Intracisternal type A particles in murine pancreatic B cells: immunocytochemical demonstration of increased antigen (p73) in genetically diabetic mice. Am J Pathol 114: 46–55

Leiter EH, Wilson GL (1988) Viral interactions with pancreatic β cells. In: Lefebvre PJ, Pipeleers (eds) The pathology of the endocrine pancreas in diabetes. Springer, Berlin Hiedelberg New York, pp 85–105

Leiter EH, Beamer WG, Shultz LD (1983) The effect of immunosuppression on streptozotocin-induced diabetes in C57BL/KsJ mice. Diabetes 32: 148–155

Leiter EH, Fewell JW, Kuff EL (1986) Glucose induces intracisternal type A retroviral gene transcription and translation in pancreatic β cells. J Exp Med 163: 87–100

Leiter EH, Le PH, Coleman DL (1987) Susceptibility to db gene and streptozotocin induced diabetes in C57BL mice: control by gender associated MHC-unlinked traits. Immunogenetics 26: 6–13

Leiter EH, Le PH, Prochazka M, Worthen SM, Huppi K (1989) Genetic and environemental control of diabetes induction by multi-dose streptozotocin in two BALB/c substrains. Diabetes Res 9: 5–10

Like AA, Rossini AA (1976) Streptozotocin-induced pancreatic insulitis: new model of diabetes mellitus. Science 193: 415–417

MacLaren NK, Neufeld M, McLaughlin JV, Tayler G (1980) Androgen sensitization of steptozotocin-induced diabetes in mice. Diabetes 29: 710–716

Magee PN (1975) *N*-nitroso compounds and related carcinogens. In: Searl CE (ed) Chemical carcinogens. American Chemical Society, Washington, DC, pp 491–509

Magee PN, Barnes JM (1956) The production of malignant primary hepatic tumors in the rat by feeding dimethylnitrosamine. Br J Cancer 10: 114–120

Mattes WB, Hartley JA, Kohn KW, Matheson DW (1988) GC-rich regions in genomes as targets for DNA alkylation. Carcinogenesis 9: 2065–2072

Mazelis AG, Albert D, Crisa C, Fiore H, Parasaram D, Franklin B, Ginsberg-Fellner F, McEvoy RC (1987) Relationship of stressful housing conditions to the onset of diabetes mellitus induced by multiple, sub-diabetogenic doses of streptozotocin in mice. Diabetes Res 6: 195–200

McEvoy RC, Andersson J, Sandler S, Hellerstrom C (1984) Mutiple low-dose streptozotocin-induced diabetes in the mouse. Evidence for stimulation of a cytotoxic cellular immune response against an insulin-producing β cell line. J Clin Invest 74: 715–722

McEvoy RC, Thomas NM, Hellerstrom C, Ginsberg-Fellner F, Moran TM (1987) Multiple low-dose steptozotocin-induced diabetes in the mouse: further evidence for involvement of an anti-B cell cytotoxic cellular autoimmune response. Diabetologia 30: 232–238

Morley JE, Kay NE, Solomon GF, Plotnikoff NP (1987) Neuropeptides: conductors of the immune orchestra. Life Sci 41: 527–544

Morrow DL, Freedman A, Craighead JE (1980) Testosterone effect on experimental diabetes mellitus in encephalomyocarditis (EMC) virus infectd mice. Diabetologia 18: 247–249

Mossman BT, Wilson GL, Ireland C, Craighead JE (1985) A diabetogenic analogue of streptozotocin with dissimilar mechanisms of action of pancreatic β cells. Diabetes 34: 602–607

Nakamura M, Nagafuchi S, Yamaguchi K, Takaki R (1984) The role of thymic immunity and insulitis in the development of streptozotocin-induced diabetes in mice. Diabetes 33: 894–900

Nakano K, Mordes JP, Handler ES, Greiner DL, Rossini AA (1988) Role of host immune system in BB/Wor rat: predisposition to diabetes resides in bone marrow. Diabetes 37: 522–525

Nerup J, Mandrup-Xoulsen T, Molvig J, Helqvist S, Wogensen L, Egeberg J (1988) Mechanisms of pancreatic β cell destruction in type 1 diabetes. Diabetes Care 11: 16–23

Nichols WK, Vann LL, Spellman JB (1981) Streptozotocin effects on T lymphocytes and bone marrow cells. Clin Exp Immunol 46: 627–632

Oldstone MBA (1988) Prevention of type 1 diabetes in nonobese diabetic mice by virus infection. Science 23: 500–502

Oschilewski M, Schwab E, Kiesel U, Opitz U, Stunkel K, Kolb-Bachofen V, Kolb H (1986) Administration of silica or monoclonal antibody to Thy-1 prevents low-dose streptozotocin-induced diabetes in mice. Immunol Lett 12: 289–294

Paik SG, Blue M, Fleischer N, Shin SI (1982a) Diabetes susceptibility of BALB/cBOM mice treated with streptozotocin. Inhibition by lethal irradition and restoration by splenic lymphocytes. Diabetes 31: 808–815

Paik SG, Michelis MA, Kim YT, Shin S (1982b) Induction of insulin dependent diabetes by streptozotocin. Inhibition by estrogens and potentiation by androgens. Diabetes 31: 724–729

Prosser PR, Karam JH (1978) Diabetes mellitus following rodenticide ingestion in man. JAMA 239: 1148–1150

Pukel C, Baquerizo H, Rabinovitch A (1988) Destruction of rat islet cell monolayers by cytokines. Synergistic interactions of interferon-γ, tumor necrosis factor, lymphotoxin, and interleukin 1. Diabetes 37: 133–136

Rakieten N (1963) Studies on the diabetogenic action of streptozotocin (NSC-37917). Cancer Chemother Rep 29: 91–103

Rossini AA, Appel M, Williams RM, Like AA (1977) Genetic influence of streptozotocin-induced insulitis and hyperglycemia. Diabetes 26: 916–920

Rossini AA, Williams RM, Appel MC, Like AA (1978a) Sex differences in the multi-dose streptozotocin model of diabetes. Endocrinology 103: 1518–1520

Rossini AA, Williams RM, Appel MC, Like AA (1978b) Complete protection from low-dose streptozotocin-induced diabetes in mice. Nature 276: 182–184

Sander J, Burke G (1971) Induktion maligner Tumoren bei Ratten durch orale Gabe von 2-Imidazolidinon und Nitrat. Krebsforschnung 75: 301–310

Sandler S, Andersson A (1981) Islet implantation into diabetic mice with pancreatic insulitis. Acta Pathol Microbiol Immunol Scand [A] 89: 107–112

Sanz N, Karam JH, Horita S, Bell GI (1986) Prevalence of insulin-gene mutations in non-insulin-dependent diabetes mellitus. N Engl J Med 314: 1322

Schwab E, Burkart V, Freytag G, Kiesel U, Kolb H (1986) Inhibition of immune mediated low-dose streptozotocin diabetes by agents which reduce vascular permeability. Immunopharmacology 12: 17–21

Schwizer RW, Leiter EH, Evans R (1984) Macrophage-mediated cytotoxicity against cultured pancreatic islet cells. Transplantation 37: 539–544

Sen WP (1973) Nitrosophyrrolidine and dimethylnitrosamine in bacon. Nature 241: 473–475

Sensi M, Pozzilli P, Ventiglia L, Doniach I, Cudworth AG (1982) Histology of the islets of Langerhans following administration of human lymphocytes into athymic mice. Clin Exp Immunol 49: 81–86

Serreze DV, Leiter EH, Worthen SM, Shultz LD (1988a) NOD marrow stem cells adoptively transfer diabetes to resistant (NOD x NON) F1 mice. Diabetes 37: 252–255

Serreze DV, Leiter EH, Kuff EL, Jardieu P, Ishizaka K (1988b) Molecular mimicry between insulin and retroviral antigen p73: development of cross reactive autoantibodies in sera of NOD and C57BL/Ks-*db*/*db* mice. Diabetes 37: 351–357

Serreze DV, Worthen SM, Leiter EH (1989) Genetic control of immunological suppressor function in BALB/c substrains: potential relation to diabetes susceptibility. Clin Exp Immunol (manuscript submitted)

Sesfontein WJ, Huster P (1966) Nitrosoamines as environmental carcinogens II. evidence for the presence of nitrosoamines in tobacco smoke condensate. Cancer Res 26: 575–583

Shiloh Y, Becker Y (1981) Kinetics of O^6- methylguanine repair in human normal and ataxia telangiectasia cell lines and correlation on repair capacity with cellular sensitivity to methylating agents. Cancer Res 41: 5114–5120

Shooter KV, Slade TA (1977) The stability of methyl and ethyl phosphotriesters in DNA in vivo. Chem Biol Interact 19: 353: 353–362

Shooter KV, Slade TA, O'Connor PJ (1977) The formation and stability of methyl phosphotriesters in the DNA of rat tissues after treatment with the carcinogen *N*,*N*-dimethylnitrosoamine. Chem Biol Interact 19: 363–374

Shultz LD, Sidman CL (1987) Genetically determined murine models of immunodeficiency. Annu Rev Immunol 5: 367–375

Sklar R, Srauss B (1980) Removal of O^6-methylguanine from DNA of normal and xeroderma pigmentosum-derived lymphoblastoid lines. Nature 289: 417–420

Stavehagen JB, Robins DM (1988) An ancient provirus has imposed androgen regulation on the adjacent mouse sex-limited protein gene. Cell 55: 247–254

Suenaga K, Yoon JW (1988) Association of β cell specific-expression of endogenous retrovirus with development of insulitis and diabetes in NOD mouse. Diabetes 37: 1722–1726

Suzuki T, Yamada T, Takao T, Fujimura T, Kawamura E, Shimizu ZM, Yamashita R, Nomoto K (1987) Diabetogenic effects of lymphocyte transfusion on the NOD or NOD nude mouse. In: Rygaard J, Brunner N, Graem N, Sprang-Thomsen M (eds) Immune-deficient animals in biomedical research. Karger, Basel, pp 112–116

Tjalve H (1983) Streptozotocin: distribution, metabolism, and mechanisms of action. Ups J Med Sci [Suppl] 39: 145–157

Uehara A, Gottschall PE, Dahl RR, Arimuri A (1987) Interleukin-1 stimulates ACTH release by an indirect action which requires endogenous corticotropin releasing factor. Endocrinology 121: 1580–1583

Wiggans RG, Woolley PV, MacDonald JS, Smythe T, Ueno W, Schein PS (1958) Phase II trial of streptozotocin, mitomycin-c, and 5-fluorouracil (SMF) in treatment of advanced pancreatic cancer. Cancer 41: 387–391

Wilander E, Boquist L (1972) Streptozotocin diabetes in the chinese hamster: blood glucose and structural changes in the first 24 hours. Horm Metab Res 4: 42–65

Wilson GL, Hartig PC, Patton NJ, LeDoux SP (1988) Mechanisms of nitrosourea-induced β cell damage: activation of poly (ADP-ribose) synthetase and cellular distribution. Diabetes 37: 213–216

Wolf J, Lilly F, Shin S (1984) The influence of genetic backoround on the susceptibility of inbred mice to streptozotocin-induced diabetes. Diabetes 33: 567–571

Yamamoto H, Uchigata Y, Okamoto H (1981) Streptozotocin and alloxan induce DNA strand breaks and poly(ADP-ribose) synthetase in pancreatic islets. Nature 294: 284–286

Yoon JW, Ray UR (1986) Perspectives on the role of viruses in insulin-dependent diabetes. Diabetes Care 8: 39–44

Yoon JW, McClintock PR, Bachurski CJ, Longstreth JD, Notkins, AL (1985) Virus induced diabetes mellitus. No evidence for immune mechanisms in the destruction of β cells by the D-variant of enchephalomyocarditis virus. Diabetes 34: 922–925

Zarbl H, Sukumar S, Arthur AV, Martin-Zanca D, Barbacid M (1985) Direct mutagenesis of Ha-*ras*-1 oncogenes by *N*-nitroso-*N*-methylurea during initiation of mammary carcinogenesis in rats. Nature 315: 382–385

Ziegler M, Ziegler B, Hehmke B, Dietz H, Hildmann W, Kauert C (1984) Autoimmune response directed to pancreatic β cells in rats induced by combined treatment with low doses of streptozotocin and complete Freund's adjuvant. Biomed Biochim Acta 43: 675–681

Ziegler M, Teneberg S, Witt S, Ziegler B, Hehmke B, Kohnert KD, Egeberg J, Karlsson KA, Lernmark A (1988) Islet β-cytotoxic monoclonal antibody against glycolipids in experimental diabetes induced by low dose streptozotocin and Freund's adjuvant. J Immunol 140: 4144–4150

Autoantigen (64000-M_r) Expression in Coxsackievirus B4-Induced Experimental Diabetes*

I. GERLING and N. K. CHATTERJEE

1 Introduction

Extensive epidemiologic observations (GAMBLE et al. 1969; GAMBLE 1980; BARRET-CONNOR 1985), many case reports, and animal studies (CRAIGHEAD 1975; NOTKINS 1977) have associated group B coxsackieviruses in the etiology of type 1, insulin-dependent diabetes mellitus (IDDM). IDDM in human patients is rare until 9 months of age and has peaks of onset at 5–8 years and again at 10–14 years of age (GAMBLE 1977). These observations are consistent with epidemiological patterns of many infections, which are prevented by maternal immunity and have peaks at the time of entry into school and at early puberty.

Although seroepidemiologic studies are too inconsistent to allow definite conclusions, most of them indicate increased titers of antibodies to coxsackievirus B4 (CB4) in newly diagnosed diabetics (GAMBLE 1977; HAZVA et al. 1980; SCHMIDT et al. 1978; ANDERSEN et al. 1977; TONIOLO et al. 1988; PALMER et al. 1982). Methodologic differences might explain the controversial results. Since diabetics produce lower titers of antibodies to CB4 following infection than matched controls (TONIOLO et al. 1988; PALMER et al. 1982), assays with different sensitivities could find increased or decreased prevalence of CB4 antibodies while comparing the same group of diabetics and controls. Another problem is the matching of controls for HLA types. The prevalence of HLA-DR3 and DR4 types is increased in IDDM patients (SVEJGAARD et al. 1983); these genotypes seem to influence the immune response, including the antibody production, to CB4 (BRUSERUD et al. 1985; SCHERNTHANER et al. 1985). This could influence the conclusions in studies where the controls are not matched for HLA-DR3 and DR4.

The reason for increased prevalence of CB4 antibodies in newly diagnosed IDDM patients remains elusive. The immunoglobulin M (IgM) nature of the response indicates a recent infection (SCHERNTHANER et al., 1985). Even though

Wadsworth Center for Laboratories and Research, New York State Department of Health, Empire State Plaza, P.O. Box 509 Albany, NY 12201-0509, USA
* This work was supported by grants AM33054 from the National Institute of Health and HRI 815-3506F from the Biomedical Research Support, New York State Department of Health

experiments in animals (MONTGOMERY and LORIA 1988) indicate a correlation between the diabetic milieu and immune response to CB4, this is probably not the case in humans since no difference in metabolic control was found between CB4 IgM positive and CB4 IgM negative IDDM patients (SCHERNTHANER et al. 1985).

If CB4 infection is an important factor in the etiology of IDDM, it is important to recognize that the virus-specific antibody tests will not distinguish between diabetogenic and nondiabetogenic viruses. It is also important to consider that no, low, or even late CB4 antibody response is expected in individuals most seriously affected by the virus infection since antibodies are a marker for a successful immune response to the infection. Finally, experiments in animals indicate an increased diabetogenic potential of CB4 if the virus is injected in conjunction with other diabetogenic viruses or diabetes-inducing drugs (TONIOLO et al. 1980; JORDAN et al. 1985). Immunological tests that are currently available may therefore be poor indicators of a diabetogenic CB4 infection.

2 CB4-Induced Experimental Diabetes

Experimental studies on CB4-induced diabetes were performed in mice (YOON et al. 1978, 1979; WEBB and MADGE 1980) since the virus seems to grow and readily adapt in several strains of mice. Diabetogenic strains of CB4 were isolated from human source, e.g., the pancreas of a child who died after abrupt onset of diabetic ketoacidosis (YOON et al. 1979) or developed by serial passages of prototype virus in beta cell-enriched cultures (YOON et al. 1978).

The possibility of developing diabetogenic strains from nondiabetogenic CB4 indicates either a high rate of mutation in the virus genome or heterogeneity in the virus particles within a single isolate or strain. Experimental evidence support both mechanisms. A rate of mutation as high as 10^{-4} was suggested by studies on antigenic variation using CB4 monoclonal antibodies (PRABHAKAR et al. 1982). The CB4 virus we have used originated from a strain (Edwards) which was isolated from myocardial tissue of an infant dying of generalized coxsackievirus infection, focal necrosis, and inflammation of the pancreas (KIBRICK and BENIRSCHKE 1958) and then passaged three times in vivo in mouse pancreas (WEBB et al. 1976). Three clones were selected from this passaged virus by repeated plaque purification. The three clones differed from the original isolate and from each other with respect to accumulation of CB4 antigen in islets and acinar cells, as well as in their ability to change blood glucose and plasma amylase content after injection in two different mice strains (HARTIG et al. 1983; HARTIG and WEBB 1983). We have used one of these clones called E2. E2 was later found to separate into two distinct populations of particles with different densities $\rho = 1.34$ and 1.29) (CHATTERJEE et al. 1988). These two populations showed differences in infectivity and diabetogenicity: the less infective population ($\rho = 1.29$) appeared to be more diabetogenic.

Not all strains of mouse are susceptible to the diabetogenic effect of CB4. With a few possible exceptions, the same strain may be susceptible to diabetes induction by different diabetogenic CB4 strains (WEBB and MADGE 1980), as well as by encephalomyocarditis virus, another diabetogenic picornavirus (YOON et al. 1978). Susceptibility to CB4-induced diabetes is inherited as an autosomal recessive trait (WEBB and MADGE 1980). Diabetes-resistant strains are also affected by the diabetogenic potential of the virus, but the effect may not be strong enough to develop diabetes, because CB4 infection of such a strain after injection with a subdiabetogenic dose of streptozotocin leads to hyperglycemia (WEGNER et al. 1985). The virus replicates to the same extent in the pancreas of both diabetes-prone and diabetes-resistant mice, but an inverse relationship between the effect of CB4 infection on exocrine and endocrine pancreas was reported. Susceptible mice had less severe acinar pancreatitis than resistant mice (WEBB and MADGE 1980), while staining for CB4 antigens produced much stronger stain in islets from susceptible mice than from resistant mice (HARTIG et al. 1983).

We have studied the kinetics of diabetes development in susceptible mice after infection with CB4-E2 virus. The incidence of diabetes appears to follow a bimodal distribution: 53% diabetes at 1 week postinfection (p.i.), the incidence decreasing to 26% at 3 weeks p.i. and then sharply increasing to 100% diabetes at 4 weeks p.i. (GERLING et al. 1989). The exact pathogenic mechanism for the induction of diabetes in this system is currently unknown. Our studies are concentrated on three possible mechanisms: (1) direct cytolytic infection of beta cells, (2) triggering of autoimmunity, and (3) functional impairment of beta cells by persistent infection.

3 Cytolytic Infection

CB4 virus can infect, replicate, and lyse certain tissue culture cells to produce infectious virus. We detected large amounts of infectious virus in the pancreatic islets of E2-infected mice at 72 h p.i.; however, the virus was barely detectable at 1 week p.i. and not at all later (CHATTERJEE et al. 1985; GERLING et al. 1989). It should be pointed out that the infected beta cells contained a fair amount of viral RNA at 6 weeks and 8 weeks p.i. (CHATTERJEE and NEJMAN 1988). We think that cytolytic infection causes diabetes observed at 1 week p.i. since virus replication is maximum at 72 h p.i. (GERLING et al. 1989). This is also supported by the results of a previous histochemical study (HARTIG et al. 1983) in which the authors detected a few necrotic endocrine cells, viral antigens in the beta cells, and extensive degranulation of the cells at 72 h p.i. in CB4 E2-infected mice.

Hypoglycemia was detected in some virus-infected mice at 72 h p.i. (HARTIG and WEBB 1983; CHATTERJEE et al. 1985). This may be due to an increased glucose sensitivity of the islets since both glucose-stimulated insulin release and residual insulin content after release increased in islets isolated from mice at 72 h p.i. (GERLING et al. 1988). Total protein and insulin synthesis decreased (CHATTERJEE et al. 1985) with a decrease in poly(A)-containing total mRNA, but not insulin mRNA (CHATTERJEE and NEJMAN 1988). The reason for the decrease in total mRNA, and not insulin mRNA, could be due to longer half-life of the latter. Another interesting observation is the increased synthesis of a protein presumably glyceraldehyde-3-phosphate dehydrogenase in the islets at 72 h p.i. (GERLING et al. 1988), which could be important since this enzyme may be involved in the regulation of glucose-stimulated insulin release (HEDESKOV 1980).

4 Autoimmunity

Synthesis of a second islet protein, 64000-M_r (64 kDa) increased at 72 h p.i. (GERLING et al. 1988). This protein could only be immunoprecipitated with sera from IDDM patients, containing antibodies to the IDDM associated 64 kDa islet cell autoantigen (BAEKKESKOV et al. 1982). Detection of mouse antigen with human 64 kDa autoantibodies is not surprising since several studies showed these antibodies to be species nonspecific (BAEKKESKOV and LERNMARK 1982; GERLING et al. 1986). Antibodies to the 64 kDa autoantigen precede the onset of IDDM in humans and in spontaneously diabetic BB rats (BAEKKESKOV et al. 1984, 1987), and it was suggested that the 64 kDa protein is a major target antigen in an autoimmune process leading to the development of IDDM. It was therefore of interest to determine if CB4 E2-infected mice developed autoantibodies to the 64 kDa antigen. Sera, collected from groups of 9–19 mice at different times p.i. were examined for the presence of such antibodies by immunoprecipitation. The incidence of 64 kDa antibodies was 11% (1 of 9) in noninfected CD-1 mice, which increased steadily with the time of infection to 89% at 4 weeks p.i. (GERLING et al. 1989).

If the infection is considered to be a trigger of this autoantibody response, one possible mechanism would be that the increased 64 kDa autoantigen expression in conjunction with possible aberrant expression of MHC Class II antigens in the islets and beta cells (BOTTAZZO et al. 1985) would make the cells to function as antigen-presenting cells. This would trigger an immune reaction against the 64 kDa antigen. At present we cannot rule out the possibility of molecular mimicry or cross-reaction between the 64 kDa antigen and CB4 epitopes as a mechanism for 64 kDa autoantibody induction. It is very unlikely that the 64 kDa antigen is a viral-encoded protein since no protein of this molecular weight was detected in CB4-infected tissue culture cells (CHATTERJEE and TUCHOWSKI 1981). Furthermore, noninfected control mice also contain this antigen.

The incidence of diabetes at 6 weeks p.i. was quite low, 20%–25%, in animals that were bled once between 72 h p.i. and 2 weeks p.i. compared with that of 80% in animals not bled at all (GERLING et al. 1989). Prevention of diabetes by blood removal in young prediabetic BB rats was reported (YALE et al. 1988), which was correlated with changes in several T-lymphocyte subsets. The exact mechanism that lowers diabetes in E2-infected mice is currently unknown.

5 Persistent Infection

Persistent infection by coxsackie B viruses is becoming increasingly evident in recent studies (BOWLES et al. 1986; MCCARTNEY et al. 1986; CHATTERJEE and NEJMAN 1988). In our E2 virus-infected mice, even though we could not detect infectious virus in the pancreatic islets after 1 week, a fair amount of RNA was detected by molecular hybridization at 6 weeks and 8 weeks p.i. (CHATTERJEE and NEJMAN 1988), strongly suggesting a persistent infection in the beta cells. These persistently infected islets of 6 weeks p.i. showed a significant reduction in glucose-stimulated insulin release and residual islet insulin content after release (GERLING et al. 1988). Both poly(a)-containing total mRNA and insulin mRNA levels were significantly reduced (CHATTERJEE and NEJMAN 1988). Protein synthesis measured by ^{35}S-methionine incorporation in islet cultures also decreased. A decrease in the synthesis of several proteins at 72 h p.i. and virtually all proteins at 6 weeks was apparent (GERLING et al. 1988). In another study (CHATTERJEE et al. 1989) the pancreatic somatostatin content and somatostatin mRNA supply appeared significantly depressed in islets of the infected mice. Persistent virus infection has been proposed to distort specialized cell functions and to induce diabetes in lymphocytic choriomeningitis virus-infected mice (OLDSTONE et al. 1984). In our study, altered glucose-stimulated insulin release in the islets of E2-infected mice most likely resulted from such persistent infection. It is also possible that binding of 64 kDa antibodies to beta cells alters the sensitivity of the islets to glucose since incubation of beta cells with diabetic immunoglobulin inhibited glucose-stimulated insulin release (KANATSUNA et al. 1983).

6 Concluding Remarks

Different methods have successfully been used to generate diabetogenic CB4 strains. The most important step seems to be passage of the virus in beta cells either in vitro or in vivo to select for beta cell-trophic particles which may be very rare in wild-type virus. Diabetogenic CB4 strains developed by different methods produce similar effects in susceptible mice. Nevertheless, a few differences between them exist. Therefore, the possibility that different strains may cause diabetes by different mechanisms cannot be ruled out.

The apparent biphasic nature of E2 virus-induced diabetes suggests the possibility of a fast-developing disease at 72 h to 2 weeks p.i. and a slow-developing one at 4 weeks which could be induced by different mechanisms. As previously stated, the fast-developing diabetes is most likely due to a lytic infection in the pancreas. The disease appears simultaneously with or shortly after infectious virus can be detected in the islets. Both persistent infection and autoimmunity are slow processes, these probably do not induce the disease seen very early at 72 h p.i.

Our studies are predominantly on the slow-developing diabetes that resembles IDDM in humans. Like the human disease, in our mouse model, the interval between virus infection (triggering event) and diabetes development is long. Furthermore, 64 kDa autoantibodies also appear before the onset, emphasizing the role of autoimmunity in this model. It is unlikely that lytic infection causes slow diabetes since infectious virus disappears from the islets of the diabetic animals. Persistent infection appears to play an important role in slow diabetes and probably leads to functional impairment in the remaining beta cells.

A promising area of investigation is the prevention of slow diabetes by blood withdrawal. Our preliminary study shows a dramatic reduction in the incidence of diabetes soon after virus infection. It will be interesting to discover whether the reduced diabetes incidence in E2 virus-infected mice occurs via immune correction.

Acknowledgment. We thank Nancy Miller for her expert assistance during the preparation of this manuscript.

References

Andersen OO, Christy M, Arnung K, Buschard K, Christau B, Kromann H, Nerup J, Platz P, Ryder LP, Svejgaard A, Thomsen M (1977) Viruses and diabetes. In: Bajaj JS(ed) Diabetes. Excerpta Medica, Amsterdam, pp 294–298

Baekkeskov S, Lernmark A (1982) Rodent islet cell antigens recognized by antibodies in sera from diabetic patients. Acta Biol Med Ger 4: 111–115

Baekkeskov S, Nielsen JH, Marner B, Bilde T, Ludvigsson J, Lernmark A (1982) Autoantibodies in newly diagnosed diabetic children immunoprecipitate human pancreatic islet cell proteins. Nature 298: 167–169

Baekkeskov S, Dyrberg T, Lernmark A (1984) Autoantibodies to a 64-kilodalton islet cell protein precede the onset of spontaneous diabetes in the BB rat. Science 224: 1348–1350

Baekkeskov S, Landin M, Kristensen JK, Srikanta S, Bruining GJ, Poulsen TM, Beaufort C, Soeldner JS, Eisenbarth G, Lindgren F, Sundquist G, Lernmark A (1987) Antibodies to a 64,000 M_r human islet cell antigen precede the clinical onset of insulin-dependent diabetes. J Clin Invest 79: 926–934

Barret-Connor E (1985) Is insulin-dependent diabetes mellitus caused by coxsackievirus B infection? A review of the epidemiologic evidence. Rev Infect Dis 7: 207–215

Bottazzo GF, Dean BM, McNally JM, Mackay EH, Swift PGF, Gamble DR (1985) In situ characterization of autoimmune phenomena and expression of HLA molecules in the pancreas in diabetic insulitis. N Engl J Med 313: 353–360

Bowles NE, Olsen EGJ, Richardson PJ, Archard LC (1986) Detection of coxsackie B virus-specific RNA sequences in myocardial biopsy samples from patients with myocarditis and dilated cardiomyopathy. Lancet 1: 1120–1123

Bruserud O, Jervell J, Thorsby E (1985) HLA-DR3 and DR4 control T-lymphocyte responses to mumps and coxsackie B4 virus: studies on patients with Type 1 (insulin-dependent) diabetes and healthy subjects. Diabetologia 28: 420–426

Chatterjee NK, Nejman C (1988) Insulin mRNA content in pancreatic beta cells of coxsackievirus B4-induced diabetic mice. Mol Cell Endocrinol 55: 193–202

Chatterjee NK, Tuchowski C (1981) Comparison of capsid polypeptides of group B coxsackieviruses and polypeptide synthesis in infected cells. Arch Virol 70: 255–269

Chatterjee NK, Haley TM, Nejman C (1985) Functional alterations in pancreatic B cells as a factor in virus-induced hyperglycemia in mice. J Biol Chem 260: 12786–12791
Chatterjee NK, Nejman C, Gerling I (1988) Purification and characterization of a strain of coxsackievirus B4 of human origin that induces diabetes in mice. J Med Virol 26: 57–69
Chatterjee NK, Gerling I, Nejman C (1989) Pancreatic D-cell disorder in Coxsackie-virus B4-induced diabetic mice. Mol Cell Endocrinol 67: 39–45
Craighead JE (1975) The role of viruses in the pathogenesis of pancreatic diseases and diabetes mellitus. Prog Med Virol 19: 161–214
Gamble DR (1977) Viruses and diabetes: an overview with special reference to epidemiological studies. In: Bajaj JS (ed) Diabetes. Excerpta Medica, Amsterdam, pp 283–293
Gamble DR (1980) The epidemiology of insulin dependent diabetes, with particular reference to the relationship of virus infection to its etiology. Epidemiol Rev 2: 49–70
Gamble DR, Kinsley ML, Fitzgerald MG, Bolton R, Taylor KW (1969) Viral antibodies in diabetes mellitus. Br Med J 3: 627–630
Gerling I, Baekkeskov S, Lernmark A (1986) Islet cell and 64K autoantibodies are associated with plasma IgG in newly diagnosed insulin-dependent diabetic children. J Immunol 137: 3782–3785
Gerling I, Nejman C, Chatterjee NK (1988) Effect of coxsackievirus B4 infection in mice on expression of 64,000 M_r autoantigen and glucose sensitivity of islets before development of hyperglycemia. Diabetes 37: 1419–1425
Gerling I, Chatterjee NK, Nejman C (1990) Development of 64,000-M_r autoantibodies in coxsackievirus B4-induced hyperglycemic mice. (submitted)
Hartig PC, Webb SR (1983) Heterogeneity of a human isolate of coxsackie B4: biological differences. J Infect 6: 43–48
Hartig PC, Madge GE, Webb SR (1983) Diversity within a human isolate of coxsackie B4: relationship to viral-induced diabetes. J Med Virol 11: 23–30
Hazva DK, Singh R, Wahal PK, Gupta MK, Jain NK, Elhence BR (1980) Coxsackie antibodies in young Asian diabetics. Lancet 1: 877
Hedeskov CJ (1980) Mechanism of glucose-induced insulin secretion. Physiol Rev 60: 442–507
Jordan GW, Bolton V, Schmidt NJ (1985) Diabetogenic potential of coxsackie B viruses in nature. Arch Virol 86: 213–221
Kanatsuna T, Baekkeskov S, Lernmark A, Ludvigsson J (1983) Immunoglobulin from insulin-dependent diabetic children inhibits glucose-induced insulin release. Diabetes 32: 520–524
Kibrick S, Benirschke K (1958) Severe generalized disease (encephalohepatomyocarditis) occurring in the newborn period and due to infection with coxsackievirus group B. Pediatrics 22: 857–875
McCartney RA, Banatvala JE, Bell EJ (1986) The routine use of μ-antibody capture ELISA for the serological diagnosis of coxsackie B virus infection. J Med Virol 19: 205–212
Montgomery LB, Loria RM (1988) The use of coxsackievirus B4 to probe immunodeficiencies associated with hereditary and overt diabetes mellitus. Diabetes 7: 209A
Notkins AL (1977) Virus-induced diabetes mellitus. Arch Virol 54: 1–17
Oldstone MBA, Southern P, Rodriguez M, Lampert PW (1984) Virus persists in beta cells and islets of Langerhans and is associated with chemical manifestation of diabetes. Science 224: 1440–1444
Palmer JP, Cooney MK, Ward RH, Hansen JA, Brodsky JB, Ray CG, Crossley JR, Asplin CM, Williams RH (1982) Reduced coxsackie antibody titers in type 1 (insulin-dependent) diabetic patients presenting during an outbreak of coxsackie B3 and B4 infection. Diabetologia 22: 426–429
Prabhakar BS, Haspel MV, McClintock PR, Notkins AL (1982) High frequency of antigenic variants among naturally occurring human coxsackie B4 virus isolates identified by monoclonal antibodies. Nature 300: 374–376
Schernthaner G, Scherbaum W, Borkenstein M, Banatvala JE, Bryant J, Schober E, Mayr WR (1985) Coxsackie-B-Virus specific IgM responses, complement fixing islet-cell antibodies HLA-DR antigens and C-peptide secretion in insulin-dependent diabetes mellitus. Lancet 2: 630–632
Schmidt WAK, Brade L, Munterfering H, Klein M (1978) Course of coxsackie B antibodies during juvenile diabetes. Med Microbiol Immunol (Berl) 164: 291–298
Svejgaard A, Platz P, Ryder LP (1983) HLA and disease 1982-a survey. Immunol Rev 70: 193–218
Toniolo A, Onodera T, Yoon JW, Notkins AL (1980) Induction of diabetes by cumulative environmental insults from viruses and chemicals. Nature 288: 383–385
Toniolo A, Federico G, Basolo F, Onodera T (1988) Diabetes mellitus. In: Bendinelli M, Friedman H (ed) Coxsackieviruses–a general update. Plenum, New York, pp 351–382
Webb SR, Madge GE (1980) The role of host genetics in the pathogenesis of coxsackievirus infection in the pancreas of mice. J Infect Dis 141: 47–54

Webb SR, Loria RM, Kibrick S (1976) Susceptibility of mice to group B coxsackievirus is influenced by the diabetic gene. J Exp Med 143: 1239–1248

Wegner U, Kewitsch A, Madauss M, Dohner L, Zuhlke H (1985) Hyperglycemia in Balb/c mice after pretreatment with an subdiabetogenic dose of streptozotocin and subsequent infection with a coxsackie B4 strain. Biomed Biochim Acta 44: 21–27

Yale JF, Grose M, Seemayer TA, Marliss EB (1988) Diabetes prevention in BB rats by frequent blood withdrawal started at a young age. Diabetes 37: 327–333

Yoon JW, Onodera T, Notkins AL (1978) Virus-induced diabetes mellitus: beta cell damage and insulin dependent hyperglycemia in mice infectiod with coxsackievirus B4. J Exp Med 148: 1068–1080

Yoon JW, Austin M, Onodera T, Notkins AL (1979) Virus-induced diabetes mellitus. Isolation of a virus from the pancreas of a child with diabetic ketoacidosis. N Engl J Med 300: 1173–1179

Effects of Rubella Virus Infection on Islet Function*

E. J. RAYFIELD

1 Introduction

Viruses have been linked to the subsequent development of diabetes mellitus for at least 90 years (HARRIS 1899). The evidence to support environmental factors comes from a variety of studies including case reports in the literature, especially in regard to the congenital rubella syndrome (GINSBERG-FELLNER et al. 1985). The association of diabetes mellitus with the congenital rubella syndrome (CRS) provides the most compelling data that viruses may be directly accountable for the later onset of diabetes (RAYFIELD and ISHIMURA 1987). This chapter will first review data from human studies and then present evidence from animal models to support an association of CRS with diabetes mellitus. This is a logical sequence since it was the observations from the human studies which prompted the development of the animal models.

2 Human Studies

In an initial report in 1949, Hay noted one child with diabetes among 100 children with CRS (HAY 1949). MENSER et al. (1967) cited a second patient in a 25-year follow-up of 50 patients with CRS in New South Wales (MENSER et al. 1967). Continued observation led to subsequent papers by Menser and colleagues in which further cases were included, and a frequency of 40% was calculated from the development of diabetes in patients with CRS (FORREST et al. 1969, 1971; MENSER et al. 1974, 1978). A series of patients studied in New York has revealed the incidence of diabetes or impaired glucose tolerance to be 12% (RUBINSTEIN et al. 1982). Interestingly, strains of rubella virus seem to result in less

Clinical Professor of Medicine, Mount Sinai School of Medicine Adjunct Professor, Laboratory of Medical Biochemistry Rockefeller University, New York, NY

* This work was supported in part by grants from the National Institutes of Health (NIADDK 35003) and a grant in honor of Dr. Gerald J. Friedman

Current Topics in Microbiology and Immunology, Vol. 156

abnormalities on fetuses in Japan than in the US (Kono et al. 1985). Therefore, variations in the frequency of CRS as well as subsequent diabetes may indicate subtle genetic differences in the strains of the virus from country to country (Kono et al. 1985). Of note, some (Monif et al. 1965), but not all (Singer et al. 1967) children in whom autopsies have been performed have been found to have persistent rubella infection in their pancreatic tissue. This persistent infection results in the later impairment of insulin secretion.

CRS results in a variety of clinical abnormalities including intrauterine growth retardation, sensorineural deafness, mental retardation, patent ductus arteriosus, pulmonic stenosis, and cataracts with micropthalmia and retinopathy (Cooper 1985). In addition to diabetes mellitus (the most common of the delayed stigmata of rubella), autoimmune thyroid disease (Unterwood and Van Wyk 1981), Addison's disease (Schopfer et al. 1982) and growth hormone deficiency (Preece et al. 1977) have all been cited.

Genetic studies reveal that patients with CRS and type 1 diabetes have a significantly increased frequency of HLA DR3 and a significantly decreased frequency of DR2 (Rubinstein et al. 1982). There was also an increased frequency of HLA DR4 that was not statistically significant. It was felt that the findings with DR4 reflect an increased prevalence of this antigen in the Hispanic population in general (Rubinstein et al. 1982).

That the endocrine dysfunction in CRS might be the consequence of autoimmunity was suggested by the findings in 1984 of an increased prevalence of islet cell surface antibodies (ICSA) in 21% of the CRS study population in New York in addition to 50%–80% of patients with altered carbohydrate metabolism (Monif et al. 1965; Ginsberg-Fellner et al. 1984). Also, antithyroid microsomal and/or antithyroglobulin autoantibodies were found in 26% of patients with CRS (Ginsberg-Fellner et al. 1984, 1985). Antiadrenal antibodies were not found in the sera of 66 CRS patients tested. Of patients with CRS and type 1 diabetes 13% also exhibited insulin autoantibodies in comparison with less than 1% of the control population and 49% of new onset type 1 patients(McEvoy et al. 1986). The patients with both CRS and type 1 diabetes also tend to be ICSA positive, but no clear association with the DR3 or DR4 haplotype has been found.

Although most patients with CRS and type 1 diabetes have decreased circulating insulin levels, 18.4% of CRS patients have hyperinsulinemia. Of 17 patients who were hyperinsulinemic at the time of the initial study, three subsequently developed hypoinsulinemia; each of these three are DR3 and DR4 and have ICSA (Ginsberg-Fellner et al. 1987).

T4 (helper)/T8 (suppressor) lymphocyte studies performed in two series of patients with CRS reveal that these ratios are decreased in one half (Ginsberg-Fellner et al. 1987) to two thirds (Rabinowe et al. 1986) of each group. One of the CRS patients in each of these studies also had type 1 diabetes mellitus.

The striking nonendocrine clinical stigmata of CRS account for why the association with type 1 diabetes is not contested. The diabetes or impaired glucose tolerance that occurs may not appear until age 10–30. In contrast to CRS, other viruses implicated in human type 1 diabetes, such as coxsackie virus

B4, may frequently go unnoticed as an asymptomatic infection. In addition, the autoimmune features occurring concommitantly with CRS are very similar to those of type 1 diabetes without CRS. The current rubella vaccination programs have greatly diminished the incidence of CRS, thereby reducing the availability of patients in whom the natural history of human CRS may be studied. For these reasons it became important to develop animal models of rubella virus-induced β cell dysfunction.

3 Animal Studies

Rubella virus infection has been documented in rhesus monkeys, (PARKMAN et al. 1965; OXFORD 1967), ferrets (COTLIER et al. 1968), rats (AVILA et al. 1973; KONO et al. 1969), hamsters (COTLIER et al. 1968), and rabbits (MENSER et al. 1978; RAYFIELD et al. 1986), but not in mice. The first report of an animal model designed specifically to assess whether rubella virus infection would lead to β cell damage was described byMENSER et al. (1978). In this study, pregnant white rabbits were injected intravenously with a rubella virus inoculum grown in an RK13 rabbit-kidney continuous cell line while other rabbits were sham innoculated with diluent. This virus was derived from the kidney of a child with CRS who died at age 2 months. Offspring, delivered either spontaneously or by caesarean section, did not exhibit hyperglycemia. Electron microscopic examination of the pancreas showed β cell degranulation and swelling of mitochondria and Golgi apparatus.

3.1 Hamster Model for Neonatal Rubella Virus-Induced Diabetes

In 1986 we reported an animal model for rubella virus-induced diabetes (YOON et al. 1984).

3.1.1 Materials and Methods

3.1.1.1 Animals and Virus Preparation

Male LVG strain golden Syrian hamsters 7–10 days old (Charles River Breeding Laboratories, Wilmington, MA) were used. The vaccine strain (RA 27/3) of rubella virus was serially passaged five times (P5) in monolayer cultures enriched for pancreatic beta cells prepared from pancreata of neonatal hamsters (BOTTAZZO et al. 1974). It was necessary to adapt the virus for growth in hamster β cells to develop a diabetogenic varient of rubella for the hamster model. The hamsters were inoculated intraperitoneally (i.p.) with 10^5 plaque-forming units of the P5 variant or sham inoculated with phosphate buffered saline. Sodium pentobarbital was used to anesthetize the hamsters, and samples of blood were obtained by cardiac puncture. All hamsters inoculated with the P5 variant converted from no detectable virus antibodies to antibody titers exceeding 40. In order to isolate the virus, pancreas and lung were asepctically removed, washed extensively, homogenized and assayed for infectious virus.

3.1.1.2 Microscopy

Sequential samples of histologic sections of pancreas were obtained. They were rapidly frozen 7, 14, and 21 days after inoculation with virus or diluent, stained with hematoxylin and eosin, and islets were examined for size and mononuclear cell infiltrate.

3.1.1.3 Immunofluorescent Staining

Sections of pancreas from control and rubella virus infected hamsters were obtained 7 days after infection and a double-label flourescent antibody technique was employed to determine the presence of viral antigen in the beta cells by the simultaneous staining of cells with rubella antigen as well as those containing insulin (BOTTAZZO et al. 1974). The individual interpreting the immunofluorescent sections was unaware of whether the section originated from the control or experimental group.

3.1.1.4 Islet Cell Antibodies

Pancreata from five normal SJL/J mice were removed, fixed with Bouin's solution, cut into 4-μ sections and placed on slides. Serial dilutions of 20 sera from infected animals at 3–4 weeks following infection were incubated with pancreatic tissues for 2 h at room temperature. Then, 20 μl of a 1:20 dilution of fluorescein isothiocyanate (FITC)-labeled rabbit antihamster IgG was placed on the slides and incubated at 4°C overnight. After serial washing procedures, the specimens were inspected under a fluorescent microscope (YOON et al. 1984; JUAN and AVRUSKIN 1971).

3.1.1.5 Metabolic Studies

Each experiment with rubella virus-infected hamsters and sham-inoculated controls was performed twice using 20 animals in each group. Samples were obtained weekly for serum glucose and insulin levels measured 60 min after i.p. glucose administration (200 mg/100 g body weight).

3.1.2 Results

3.1.2.1 Body Weights

Body weights increased progressively throughout the 15 weeks of study. The control and experimental groups were very similar.

3.1.2.2 *Virus Isolation*

Rubella virus was isolated 7 days after injection from the lung and pancreas, but not the sera of all 10 hamsters tested. Virus titers in the lung ranged from 3.6×10^3 to 3.0×10^4 pfu/gram of tissue; titers in pancreas ranged from 4.0×10^2 to 1.8×10^3 pfu/gram of tissue.

3.1.2.3 *Histopathological Studies*

From each randomly selected sample of pancreas 9 of 16 islets were studied. Control islets were normal histologically. On day 14 after rubella virus inoculation, islets exhibited early evidence of inflammation. At 21 days following infection, 35.4% of islets from infected hamsters exhibited a mononuclear cell infiltrate.

3.1.2.4 *Immunofluorescent Studies*

Rubella virus antigens were detected in the beta cells isolated 14–21 days after infection by indirect immunofluorescent techniques in 8 out of 10 hamsters tested.

3.1.2.5 *Islet Cell Antibodies*

Pancreatic islet autoantibodies were measured in sera screened at 21–32 days following infection. In the experimental group 8 of 20 sera obtained from different animals were positive for islet cell antibodies (Rayfield et al. 1986).

3.1.2.6 *Metabolic Studies*

Serum glucose levels in the groups infected with rubella virus were significantly ($P < 0.001$) greater than control values 1 h following glucose administration at all time points over the 15-week study period. Mean glucose values ($\pm$ SEM) varied between 270 ± 60 mg/dl and 345 ± 70 mg/dl (Fig. 1). Serum insulin levels were significantly lower 1 h after glucose challenge in the experimental group than in the control group ($P < 0.001$) at every time point during the study (Fig. 2); (Rayfield et al. 1986).

3.1.3 Conclusions

When 7- to 10-day-old neonatal hamsters were infected with the P5 variant of rubella virus, hyperglycemia, hypoinsulinemia, insulinitis, and positive immunofluorescence for rubella viral antigen in beta cells developed. The availability of an effective rubella virus vaccine and the limitations placed on human clinical research present major problems in investigations of CRS in humans. Therefore, the findings in the neonatal golden Syrian hamster model which closely mimic human CRS are welcome.

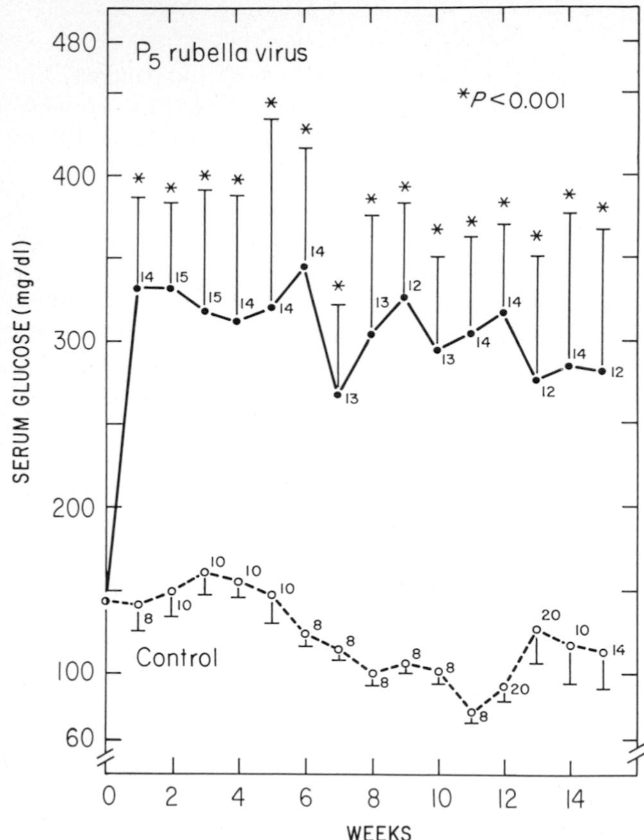

Fig. 1. Weekly serum glucose levels ($\pm$ SEM) in postglucose (200 mg/100 g body weight i.p.) over 15-week study period. $P < 0.001$ for experimental group compared with control group for respective week using students t-test for unpaired samples. *Values next to mean* indicate numbers of animals in each group

3.2 Hamster Model for Intrauterine Rubella Virus-Induced Diabetes

We also performed a preliminary study to assess intrauterine infection of hamsters with 1×10^5 pfu of the P5 variant of rubella virus in 15 female hamsters who were inoculated with virus on the 5th day of pregnancy. Following anesthesia, hamster uteri were surgically exposed under a dissecting microscope, and each side was injected with virus. Control hamsters were sham injected into the uterine cavity with diluent.

Three females aborted and an additional two died in labor. Examination of the fetuses of one of the hamsters that died in labor revealed seven embryos that were underdeveloped. The uterus of the second female contained six fetuses, one of which was underdeveloped, one was missing one hind limb (see Fig. 3), and one was without both hind limbs.

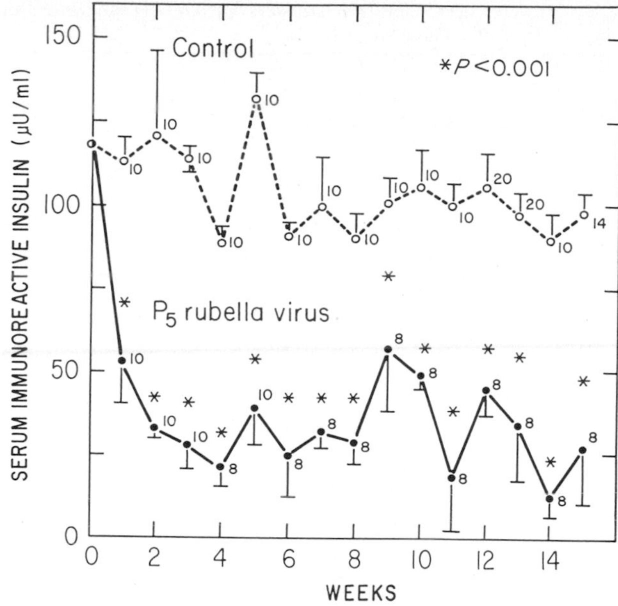

Fig. 2. Weekly serum insulin levels ($\pm$ SEM) 1 h postglucose (200 mg/100 g body weight i.p.) over 15-week study period. $P < 0.001$ for experimental group compared with control group for respective week. *Value next to mean* indicates number of animals in each group

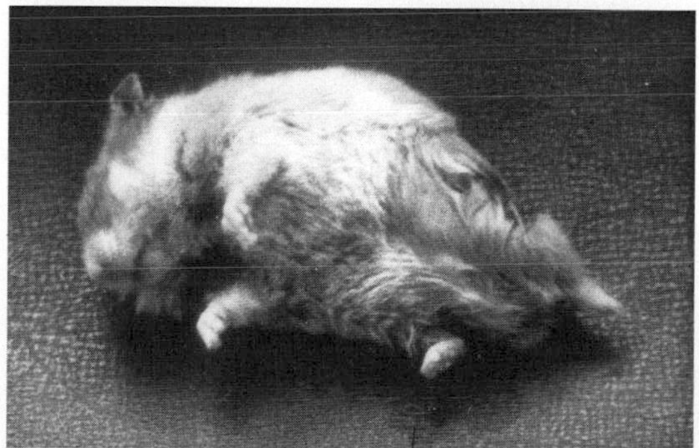

Fig. 3. Absence of hind limb in hamster infected in utero with rubella virus

Throughout the 22 days of this study with congenitally infected hamsters, there were no significant differences in weights between control and in utero infected hamsters (Table 1). There were also no differences between female and male hamsters within each group for any of the parameters measured.

At 10 days after birth, the nonfasting blood glucose levels of the infected hamsters were significantly lower ($P < 0.05$) than those of control animals. The serum insulin levels of the infected animals were significantly greater ($P < 0.05$)

Table 1. Body weight, blood glucose and serum insulin levels in hamsters congenitally infected with passaged rubella virus 8, 10, 17 and 22 days after infection

		Days after infection			
		8	10	17	22
Weight	Control (g)	10.5 ± 0.7	11.2 ± 1.3	19.5 ± 2.7	42.9 ± 1.5
	(*n*)	(3)	(6)	(3)	(6)
	Rubella (g)	8.9 ± 1.0	8.5 ± 0.7	18.7 ± 3.2	38.2 ± 2.4
	(*n*)	(3)	(5)	(3)	(5)
Blood glucose	Control (mg/dl)	96.7 ± 17.6	130.0 ± 5.2	106.7 ± 13.3	95.0 ± 6.8
	(*n*)	(3)	(6)	(3)	(6)
	Rubella (mg/dl)	88.3 ± 39.2	63.0 ± 9.7*	196.7 ± 16.7*	152.0 ± 7.3**
	(*n*)	(3)	(5)	(3)	(5)
Immuno-reactive insulin	Control (μU/ml)	32.3 ± 5.9	30.0 ± 1.4	57.3 ± 9.5	82.8 ± 13.4
	(*n*)	(3)	(6)	(3)	(6)
	Rubella (μU/ml)	168.7 ± 70.7	166.8 ± 52.8*	45.3 ± 9.2	39.8 ± 11.5*
	(*n*)	(3)	(5)	(3)	(5)

Values are means $\pm$ SEM where *n* is the number of animals in each group. * $P < 0.05$; ** $P < 0.001$

than those of control hamsters. At 17 and 22 days after birh, the nonfasting blood glucose levels of the rubella virus-infected hamsters were significantly higher ($P < 0.05$) than those of the control animals. On day 22, the serum insulin values were significantly lower than those of controls ($P < 0.05$).

These preliminary data suggest that when the P5-passaged variant of rubella virus is administered to hamsters in utero, a diabeteslike syndrome develops in the neonate associated with stigmata analogous to those seen in CRS in human.

4 Discussion

Although viruses, autoimmunity, toxins, stress, and nutritional factors may play a role in the development of insulin-dependent diabetes mellitus in a genetically susceptible host, the precise mechanisms leading to the destruction of the β cells have not been elucidated. The degree to which viruses are thought to be involved in the genesis of type 1 diabetes varies almost in a cyclical manner. Recently, several studies from Europe have shown a marked increase in the risk of developing insulin-dependent diabetes mellitus, suggesting a resurgence in the role of viruses as etiologic culprits (Rewers et al. 1987). CRS has become an important human model for type 1 diabetes (Yoon et al. 1984).

In CRS the diabetes takes 5–20 years to develop (Yoon et al. 1985), is linked to specific HLA haplotypes (Rubinstein et al. 1982), and may be associated with autoantibodies to the pancreas and the thyroid (Ginsberg-Fellner et al. 1984). As previously pointed out, the difficulties inherent in human clinical research in investigating CRS encouraged work on developing suitable animal models which would parallel the features of human CRS. The initial rabbit model did not result in hyperglycemia although there was ultrastructural evidence of β cell abnormalities. In our neonatal model, 7- to 10-day-old Syrian hamsters develop autoimmune diabetes after inoculation with a passaged variant (P5) of rubella virus. This included the presence of cytoplasmic islet cell antibodies in 8 of 20 infected animals, and rubella virus could be isolated from the pancreas 7 days after infection. Furthermore, our preliminary data show that the administration of passaged rubella virus to fetal hamsters during the first trimester of gestation results in diabetes as well as congenital anomalies similar to CRS in humans (absent hind limbs).

The failure of rubella virus to replicate in the tissue of murine strains tested to date is disappointing since immunologic studies would be simple to perform in this species. The hamster model does have the following advantages: (1) the cell line best suited for the maintenance of rubella virus, the BHK-21 line, is derived from the golden Syrian hamster (VAHERIA et al. 1967), and (2) rubella virus can be adopted into a diabetogenic variant with repeated passages in neonatal hamster β cell-enriched cultures.

What is the mechanism of rubella virus-induced diabetes? Several possibilities exist. Rubella virus could cause β cell damage by (1) directly lysing β cells (ONODERA et al. 1981), (2) promoting an autoimmune process, or (3) impairing insulin secretion as a consequence of persisting in and impairing β cell function (RAYFIELD and KELLY 1985). Since rubella virus is not extremely lytic, the first mechanism is unlikely to play a prominent role in the pathogenesis of the diabetes. An autoimmune process is supported by the presence of the resultant mononuclear cell infiltrate as well as a high frequency of islet cell (GINSBERG-FELLNER et al. 1986), thyroglobulin, and thyroid (GINSBERG-FELLNER et al. 1986) autoantibodies which occur following infection. In the hamster rubella model, islet cell antibodies occur in 8 of 20 samples measured (40%), which is certainly in keeping with an autoimmune hypothesis. Preliminary data in rat insulinoma cells does support a direct effect of rubella virus on insulin secretion (RAYFIELD and KELLY 1985). Nevertheless, the prolonged latent period of 5–20 years between in utero infection and the manifestation of clinical diabetes and the observation that 90% of the β cell mass would be required to be infected to cause hyperglycemia both weaken the importance of this mechanism.

Several hypotheses can explain the mechanism by which a virus infection may produce autoimmunity in the host. Rubella is classified as togavirus, which is an enveloped virus and is surrounded by a lipoprotein coat derived when the maturing virus buds through the host cell membrane (REINHERZ and SCHLOSSMAN 1980).

One can speculate that the virus might insert, expose, or alter antigens in the plasma membrane of the host during intracellular infection (ALLISON 1977). However, the virus might initiate an autoimmune syndrome by lysing or activating subpopulations of lymphocytes (helper or suppressor T cells) that regulate the immune response of the host (REINHERZ and SCHLOSSMAN 1980; FAUCI 1980).

5 Future Directions

Owing to the limitations imposed on human clinical research and the decreased incidence of CRS in countries where rubella vaccine is routinely administered to children, one must ask what else should be done in the CRS study group. Several studies immediately come to mind. Following the natural history of CRS with repetitive glucose tolerance tests (including insulin and C peptide levels), measurement of islet cell cytoplasmic cell surface and thyroid microsomal antibodies would be of interest. There is a subpopulation of patients with CRS who exhibit hyperinsulinemia. Will some of these individuals go on to develop hypoinsulinemia and hyperglycemia with autoantibodies? Rubella virus or a portion of it may be cultured from circulating lymphocytes of patients with CRS. If any of these individuals die from an unrelated event, tissue from pancreas, thyroid, lymph nodes, spleen, etc. can be studied for the presence of rubella viral genome.

In terms of animal models, the use of NOD and other inbred mice may be of interest if rubella virus can be adapted to murine tissue. If a neonate dies of overwhelming rubella viremia, wildvirus from this individual might be adaptable to a murine cell line. The mechanisms by which rubella virus alteration of cell membranes can lead to autoimmune events represent a fertile area of investigation.

Rubella virus remains an important potential tool for unraveling the chain of events by which a viral infection may lead to endocrine disease and autoimmunity. It is only our perseverance and ability to ask the right questions that will enable us to achieve a clearer understanding of these events.

References

Allison AC (1977) Mechanisms by which autoimmunity can be produced. In: Mendel TE, Cheer SC, Hoskins CS, McKenzie IFC, Nossal H (eds) Progress in immunology, vol III. Elsevier, North Holland, New York, p 152

Avila L, Rawls WE, Dent PB (1973) Experimental infection with rubella virus: I. acquired and congenital infection in rats. J Infect Dis 126: 585–592

Bottazzo GF, Florin-Christensen A, Doniach D (1974) Islet-cell antibodies in diabetes mellitus with autoimmune polyendocrine deficiencies. Lancet 2: 1279–1282

Cooper LZ (1985) The history of medical consequences of rubella. Rev Infect Dis 7[Suppl]: S2–S10

Cotlier E, Fox J, Bohigian G, Beaty C, Dupree A (1968) Pathogenic effects of rubella virus on embryos and newborn rats. Nature 217: 38–40

Delahunt CS, Rieser N (1967) Rubella-induced embryopathies in monkeys. Am J Obstet Gynecol 99: 580–588

Fauci AC (1980) Immunoregulation of autoimmunity. J Allergy Clin Immunol 66: 5–17

Forrest JM, Menser MA, Harley JD (1969) Diabetes mellitus and congenital rubella. Pediat 44: 445–447

Forrest JM, Menser MA, Burgess JA (1971) High frequency of diabetes mellitus in young adults with congenital rubella. Lancet 2: 332–334

Ginsberg-Fellner F, Witt ME, Yagihashi S, Dobersen MJ, Taub F, Fedun B, McEvoy RC, Roman SH, Davies TF, Cooper LZ, Rubinstein P, Notkins AL (1984) Congenital rubella-syndrome as a model for type 1 (insulin-dependent) diabetes mellitus: increased prevalance of islet cell surface antibodies. Diabetologia 27: 87–89

Ginsberg-Fellner F, Witt ME, Fedun B, Taub F, Dobersen MJ, McEvoy RC, Cooper LZ, Notkins AL, Rubinstein P (1985) Diabetes mellitus and autoimmunity in patients with congenital rubella syndrome. Rev Infect Dis 7 [Suppl 1]: S170–S175

Ginsberg-Fellner F, Fedun B, Cooper Z, Witt ME, Franklin BH, Roman SH, Rubinstein P, McEvoy RC (1987) Interrelationships of congenital rubella and type 1 insulin-dependent diabetes mellitus. In: Jaworski MA, Molnar GD, Rajotte RV, Singh B (eds) The immunology of diabetes mellitus. Elsevier, Amsterdam, pp 279–286

Harris HF (1899) A case of diabetes mellitus quickly following mumps. Boston Med Surg J 140: 465–469

Hay DR (1949) The relation of maternal rubella to congenital deafness and other abnormalities in New Zealand. NZ Med J 48: 604–608

Juan C, Avruskin TW (1971) Combined immunoassay of human growth hormone and insulin: cumulative assessment of assay performace. J Clin Endocrinol Metab 33: 150–152

Kono R, Hayakawa Y, Hibi M, Ishii K (1969) Experimental vertical transmission of rubella virus in rabbits. Lancet 1: 343–347

Kono R, Hirayama M, Sugishita C, Miyamura K (1985) Epidemiology of rubella and congenital rubella infection in Japan. Rev Infect Dis 7 [Suppl 1]: 556–563

McEvoy RC, Witt ME, Ginsberg-Fellner F, Rubinstein P (1986) Antiinsulin antibodies in children with type 1 diabetes mellitus: genetic regulation of production and presence at diagnosis before insulin replacement. Diabetes 35: 634–641

Menser MA, Dods L, Harley JD (1967) A twenty-five year follow-up of congenital rubella. Lancet 2: 1347–1350

Menser MA, Forrest JM, Honeyman MC, Burgess JA (1974) Diabetes, HLA-antigens, and congenital rubella. Lancet 2: 1508–1509

Menser MA, Forrest JM, Bransky RO (1978) Rubella infection and diabetes mellitus. Lancet 1: 57–60

Monif GRG, Avery GB, Korones SB, Sever JL (1965) Postmortem isolation of rubella virus from three children with rubella syndrome defects. Lancet 1: 723–724

Oldstone MBA, Sinha YN, Blount P, Tishon A, Rodriguez M, von Wedal R, Lampert PW (1982) Virus-induced alterations in homeostasis: alterations in differentiated functions of infected cells in vivo. Science 218: 1125–1127

Onodera T, Toniolo A, Ray UR, Jenson 4AB, Knazek RA, Notkins AL (1981) Virus-induced diabetes mellitus. XX Polyendocrinopathy and autoimmunity. J Exp Med 153: 1457–1473

Oxford JS (1967) The growth of rubella virus in small laboratory animals. J Immunol 98: 697–701

Parkman PD, Phillips PE, Krichstein RL, Meyer HM Jr (1965) Experimental rubella in the rhesus monkey. J Immunol 95: 743–752

Preece MA, Kearney PJ, Marshall WC (1977) Growth-hormone deficiency in congenital rubella. Lancet 2: 842–844

Rabinowe SL, George KL, Loughlin R, Soeldner JS, Eisenbarth GS (1986) Congenital rubella: monoclonal antibody-defined T cell abnormalities in young adults. Am J Med 81: 779–782

Rayfield EJ, Ishimura K (1987) Environmental factors and insulin-dependent diabetes mellitus. Diabetes Metab Rev 3(4): 925–957

Rayfield EJ, Kelly KJ (1985) A direct mechanism by which rubella virus impairs insulin secretion. Diabetes 34 [Suppl 1]: 68A (Abstract 271)

Rayfield EJ, Yoon JW (1981) Role of viruses in diabetes. In: Biochemistry, physiology, and pathology of the islets of Langerhans. Academic, New York, pp 427–451

Rayfield EJ, Kelly KJ, Yoon JW (1986) Rubella virus-induced diabetes in the hamster. Diabetes 35: 1278–1281

Reinherz EL, Schlossman SF (1980) Regulation of the immune response inducer and suppressor T-lymphocyte subsets in human beings. N Engl J Med 303: 370–373

Rewers M, LaPorte RE, Walczak M, Dmochowski K, Bogaczynska E (1987) Apparent epidemic of insulin-dependent diabetes mellitus in midwestern Poland 36: 106–113

Rubinstein P, Walker ME, Fedun B, Witt ME, Cooper LZ, Ginsberg-Fellner F (1982) The HLA system is congenital rubella patients with and without diabetes. Diabetes 31: 1088–1091

Schlesinger MJ, Kaarianen L (1980) Translation and processing of alpha virus proteins. In: Schlesinger RW (ed) Togaviruses. Academic, New York, pp 371–389

Schopfer K, Matter L, Flueler U, Wender E (1982) Diabetes mellitus, endocrine autoantibodies and prenatal rubella infection. Lancet 2: 159

Singer DB, Rudolf AJ, Rosenberg HS, Rawls WE, Boniu K (1967) Pathology of the congenital rubella syndrome. J Pediatr 71: 665–675

Unterwood LE, Van Wyk JJ (1981) Hormones in normal and aberrant growth. In: Williams RH (ed) Textbook of endocrinology, 6th edn. Saunders, Philadelphia, pp 1147–1184

Vaheria A, Sedurch WD, Plotkin SA (1967) Growth of rubella virus in BHK-21 cells. 1. Production, assay, and adaptation of virus. Proc Soc Exp Biol Med 125: 1086–1102

Yoon JW, Bachurski CJ, Shin SK, Archer J (1984a) Isolation, cultivation, and characterization of murine pancreatic beta cells in microculture systems. In: Phol SL, Larner J (eds) Methods in diabetes, vol 3. Wiley, New York, pp 173–184

Yoon JW, Shin SY, Bachurski CJ (1984b) Hybridomas from lymphocytes of normal mice produce monoclonal autoantibodies. Lancet 2: 641

Yoon JW, McClintock PR, Bacharski CJ, Longstreth JD, Notkins AL (1985) Virus-induced diabetes mellitus: no evidence for immune mechanisms in the destruction of β cells by the β-variant of encephalomyocarditis virus. Diabetes 34: 922–925

Monoclonal (Auto)Antibodies in Insulin-Dependent Diabetes Mellitus*

O. D. MADSEN, G. CONTREAS, and J. JØRGENSEN

1 Introduction

Insulin-dependent diabetes mellitus (IDDM) in humans, BB rats (MARLISS 1983), and nonobese diabetic (NOD) mice (MAKINO et al. 1980) is characterized by immune abnormalities leading to self-destruction of the insulin-producing islet β cells. These abnormalities have been observed in the cell-mediated as well as in the humoral immune response. Two major types of auto-antibodies have been reported, namely, islet cell cytoplasmic (ICA; BOTTAZZO et al. 1974; MACCUISH et al. 1974) and islet cell surface antibodies (ICSA; LERNMARK et al. 1978). In this chapter we will review data on experimental monoclonal antibodies to islet cells with a special emphasis on autoantibodies derived from the BB rat.

IDDM patients have a high prevalence of ICA (DELPRETE et al. 1977; LENDRUM et al. 1976), whereas such antibodies have not been detected in BB rats (MICLAREN et al. 1983). Studies suggest that antigens recognized by ICA are not β cell specific but present in all four types of islet cells. The ICA population is, however, presumably heterogeneous (SCHATZ et al. 1988), leaving the possibility that particular subpopulations may exhibit β cell specificity (i.e., insulin autoantibodies, see below). The major antigenic components recognized by ICA seem to be glycoconjugates (NAYAK et al. 1985; COLMAN et al. 1988). The apparent lack of β cell specificity has led to the hypothesis that ICA represent a secondary immune response generated by active β cell-specific destruction. Transfer studies clearly suggest that T cell immunity is involved in IDDM pathogenesis in the animal models (KOEVARY et al. 1985; BOITARD et al. 1988)

If the humoral immune response has a primary role in β cell destruction, it requires most likely the presence of a β cell-specific surface marker which for unknown reasons elicits the production of cytotoxic autoantibodies mediating cell destruction via the complement system or via antibody dependent cellular cytotoxicity (DOBERSON et al. 1980; CHARLES et al. 1983; RABINOVITCH et al. 1984; LERNMARK et al. 1984; WITT et al. 1985). In fact, ICSA have been detected in humans (LERNMARK et al. 1978), BB rats (DYRBERG et al. 1984), and NOD mice

Hagedorn Research Laboratory, DK-2820 Gentofte, Denmark

* G. CONTREAS was a recipient of a JDF fellowship, and part of the work has been supported by JDF research grant no. 188341 to OLE D. MADSEN

(reviewed by TAKEI et al. 1986), and a primary candidate for an islet cell autoantigen has been a 64-kDa protein specifically recognized by autoantibodies in sera from IDMM patients as first described by BAEKKESKOV et al. (1982). Similar antibodies were later found to be present in the BB rat (BAEKKESKOV et al. 1984) as well as in the NOD mouse (ATKINSON and MACLAREN 1988). The 64-kDa protein is likely to be a membrance protein with charge heterogenity and appears to be specifically expressed on β cells (reviewed in BAEKKESKOV and CHRISTIE 1989).

Up to now (pro) insulin remains the only well-characterized β cell-specific protein. The high prevalence of insulin auto-antibodies in IDDM patients (PALMER et al. 1983; WILKIN et al. 1985; DEAN et al. 1986), in BB rats (WILKIN et al. 1986), and in NOD mice (MARUYAMA et al. 1988) has therefore pointed towards a possible role for insulin as a β cell-specific autoantigen which marks ongoing β cell destruction. In addition, insulin immunoreactivity is selectively present on the β cell surface (KAPLAN et al. 1983; LARSSON et al. 1989). Therefore, conceptually, insulin autoantibodies can be classified as ICA as well as ICSA.

2 Experimental Monoclonal Antibodies to Islet Cells

Since the introduction of the hybridoma technique by KÖHLER and MILSTEIN (1975), extensive efforts have been made to produce monoclonal antibodies to islet cells. Several antigenic components have thus been identified (reviewed in LERNMARK 1987; POUSSIER and DAYER-MÉTROZ 1988; EISENBARTH et al. 1984; SRIKANTA and EISENBARTH 1986; EISENBARTH 1987; VARDI et al. 1987). A common feature of these experiments has been to actively immunize healthy mice with isolated islet cells, islet tumor cells, or islet cell constituents, and more recently with purified insulin granules (GRIMALDI et al. 1987), followed by selection of hybridomas for antibody binding to various islet cell components. However, only few of these monoclonal antibodies seem to be β cell specific, and any significant pathogenetic role of the corresponding antigens remains unclassified.

Another approach used was combining conventional immunization with experimentally induced diabetes (MADSEN et al. 1983b). Recently, β cell-cytotoxic monoclonal (auto)antibodies were derived from mice (ZIEGLER et al. 1988) in which diabetes had been induced by low dose streptozotocin in combination with Freund's adjuvant (ZIEGLER et al. 1984).

3 Monoclonal Antibodies to Islet Hormones

Monoclonal antibodies to a series of islet hormones have been reported, including antibodies to insulin, C peptide, proinsulin, glucagon, and somatostatin (Table 1). In general, these antibodies are highly valuable in islet cell

Table 1. Monoclonal islet hormone antibodies

Antibody	Source	Specificity	Reference
AE9 D6	Mouse IgG	Various insulins	SCHROER et al. 1983
K36aC10	Mouse IgG	Various (pro) insulins	KEILACKER et al. 1986
Mab 3	Mouse IgG1	Insulin, not proinsulin	STORCH et al. 1985
GN-ID4	Rat IgG2a	Human C peptide	MADSEN et al. 1983
GS-9A8	Mouse IgG2b	B-C junction of proinsulin	MADSEN et al. 1984
GS-4G9	Mouse IgG1		
2E6	Mouse	Proinsulin, not insulin	GRAY et al. 1987
1H1			
K79bB10	Mouse IgG1	Glucagon	WITT et al. 1987
Glu-001	Mouse IgG1	Glucagon	Novo Biolabs[a]
Som-018	Mouse IgG1	Somatostatin	Novo Biolabs[a]

The antibodies are useful islet cell typing reagents by immunocytochemistry
[a]Novo BioLabs, DK-2820 Bagsværd, Denmark

research. The proinsulin-specific antibodies GS-9A8 and GS-4G9 (reviewed in MADSEN 1987) in combination with the insulin-specific antibody, Mab 3 (STORCH et al. 1985), were instrumental in the precise mapping of the intracellular site of proinsulin sorting (ORCI et al. 1987a) and conversion in pancreatic β cells (ORCI et al. 1985, 1986, 1987b). The specificity of GN-ID4 for human (and not murine) C peptide allowed selective detection of expression of a human insulin gene when transfected into pluripotent rat insuloma cells (MADSEN et al. 1988) or when present in transgenic animals (BUCCHINI et al. 1989).

Interestingly, several of the mouse monoclonal antibodies raised against human or porcine (pro)insulins (AE9D6, K36aC10, Mab 3, GS-9A8, GS-4G9) recognize mouse (pro)insulin equally well or with slightly lower affinity (GS-4G9, GS-9A8). Despite the autoreactivity these hybridomas can be grown successfully in histocompatible mice to yield high levels of antibodies in ascites fluid (KEILACKER et al. 1986; MADSEN et al. 1983a), although preliminary evidence suggests that GS-9A8 ascites tumors induce the formation of high concentrations of anti-idiotypic antibodies (MADSEN, unpublished data). A human monoclonal autoantibody to insulin (GLEDHILL et al. 1987) was derived from a patient with anti-insulin antibodies by fusing peripheral B lymphocytes with a mouse–human heteromyeloma, SHM-D33 (TENG et al. 1983).

4 Monoclonal Autoantibodies

An obvious approach to isolating monoclonal antibodies with a pathogenetic role in IDDM would be to apply the hybridoma technique to immortalize B lymphocytes from diabetic or prediabetic patients. Despite the fact that this technique has been being used for almost 15 years in the murine system, only relatively few successful human hybridomas have been reported. Eisenbarth and coworkers published the first reports of human monoclonal islet cell autoantibody derived from a diabetic patient (EISENBARTH et al. 1982). This antibody reacted to the glucagon-producing α cell or to all islet cells by immunocytochemistry, depending on how tissue sections were processed. The fusion partner used was a human myeloma (CROCE et al. 1980) but hybridization frequencies in such experiments are low compared with those obtained when fusing mouse or rat B lymphocytes with murine myelomas (Table 2).

By using lymphocytes from the spontaneously diabetic animals, the BB rat and the NOD mouse, high yield fusions could be obtained with a greater chance to rescue and immortalize monoclonal autoantibodies which might be involved in IDDM pathogenesis.

4.1 The Diabetic NOD Mouse

Spleen cells from the NOD mouse were used to produce monoclonal autoantibodies and have given rise to an islet cell antibody, 3A4, reacting with two proteins of M_r 64 kDa and M_r 28 kDa (YOKONO et al. 1984; HARI et al. 1986). Interestingly, antisera to the 3A4 monoclonal antibody delayed the onset of diabetes when administered to prediabetic NOD mice (YOKONO et al. 1986). It remains, however, to be shown whether the 64-kDa protein recognized by 3A4 is related to the autoantigen reported previously (BÆKKESKOV et al. 1982; ATKINSON and MACLAREN 1988).

Table 2. Hybridoma fusions carried out with the aim to produce monoclonal autoantibodies to islet cells

Source of B lymphocytes	Myeloma fusion partner	Reference
Human peripheral lymphocytes (diabetic)	GM 1500[a] (human)	EISENBARTH et al. 1982
Diabetic NOD mouse spleen	FO[b] (mouse)	YOKONO et al. 1984
Diabetic C_{57}BLKsJ db/db spleen	Sp2/0-Ag14[f] (mouse)	SAI et al. 1984
Diabetic BB rat spleen	Y.3Ag 1.2.3[c] (rat) IR 983F[d] (rat)	BROGREN et al. 1986
Diabetic BB rat spleen	P3 × 63Ag 8.653[e] (mouse)	UCHIGATA et al. 1987
Prediabetic BB rat spleen	Sp2/0-Ag14[f] (mouse)	CONTREAS et al. 1988
Prediabetic BB rat spleen	P3 × 63 (mouse)	BUSE et al. 1983

References for myeloma fusion partners are as follows:
[a]CROCE et al. 1980
[b]DE ST. GROTH and SCHEIDEGGER 1980
[c]GALFRE et al. 1979
[d]BAZIN 1982
[e]KEARNEY et al. 1979
[f]SCHULMAN et al. 1978

4.2 The BB rat

Several groups have carried out direct fusions with spleen cells from diabetic or prediabetic BB rats (Table 2) with the aim to produce monoclonal islet cell antibodies (Table 3). A panel of different myelomas has been successfully applied in the various fusions (Table 2). Spleen cells were either derived from diabetic (BROGREN et al. 1986; UCHIGATA et al. 1987) or prediabetic BB rats (BUSE et al. 1983; CONTREAS et al. 1988, 1989). Screening of the various hybridoma supernatants were carried out by using islet tumor cells in cellular enzyme-linked immunoadsorbent assay (BROGREN et al. 1986; CONTREAS et al. 1988), by indirect immunofluorescence (BUSE et al. 1983), or by a combination of the two methods (CONTREAS et al. 1989). Cytotoxic islet antibodies specific for islet tumor cells were detected in ^{51}Cr release assays (USHIGATA et al. 1987).

Antibody IC2 (BROGREN et al. 1986) selectively stained the surface of isolated normal islet cells and rat islet tumor cells RINm-5F (OIE et al. 1983). Further

Table 3. Monoclonal autoantibodies derived from diabetic or prediabetic patients and animals

Antibody	Isotype	Specificity	Reference
Human			
B6	Human IgM	Pan-islet cells or A cells depending on fixation	EISENBARTH et al. 1982
NOD mouse			
3A4	Mouse IgG1	Islet cell surface anti-64-kDa and 28-kDa proteins	YOKONO et al. 1984; HARI et al. 1986
BB rat			
IC2	Rat IgM$_k$	Islet β cell surface	BROGREN et al. 1986; BUSCHARD et al. 1988
E5C2	Rat IgM	Cytotoxic islet cell surface anti-60-kDa and 68-kDa glycoprotein	UCHIGATA et al. 1987
A1G12	Rat	Islet cell cytoplasm and pannuclear membrane	BUSE et al. 1983; EISENBARTH et al. 1984
BB/TECS	Rat	Islet cell cytoplasm and thymic endocrine epithelium	BUSE et al. 1983; EISENBARTH et al. 1984
F44	Rat IgM	Islet cell cytoplasm and few scattered exocrine cells; 72-kDa antigen on western blots from several tissues	CONTREAS et al. 1988
EA512	Rat IgM	M_r 100 kDa and 23 kDa on western blots; M_r 100 kDa is endocrine specific, 23 kDa is not	CONTREAS et al. 1988
EB52	Rat IgM	Rat PP cells and few cells	CONTREAS et al. 1989
CA812	Rat IgM	Islet δ cells, but not ductal δ cells (rat, mouse, humans, monkey)	CONTREAS et al. 1989
DA39	Rat IgM	Ductal epithelium including endocrine cells in duct	CONTREAS et al. 1989
H37	Rat IgM	Pancreatic acinar cells (rat, humans, monkey)	CONTREAS et al. 1989

analyses showed that also a subpopulation of thymocytes was specifically recognized by IC2 (Poussier et al. 1986). Double staining experiments with insulin antibodies on isolated islet cells proved IC2 to be β cell specific, and the level of IC2 antigen expression correlated to the level of β cell activity (Buschard et al. 1988).

Antibody E5C2 was established from a diabetic rat and exhibited selective cytotoxicity to RINm-5F cells (Uchigata et al. 1987). Neuraminidase treatment, which removes sialic acid from glycoconjugates, enhanced indirect immunofluorescence staining of the tumor cells; the treatment was necessary to generate cytotoxicity towards isolated primary islet cells. The islet specificity of the antibody was shown by indirect staining after neuraminidase treatment of pancreas sections from rat and humans. Additionally, double-staining experiments with insulin antibodies showed surface staining of neuraminidase treated β cells. The antigenic epitope was a carbohydrate moiety, Galβ1-4GlcNAc-R, and the antigen was identified as glycoproteins of M_r 60 kDa and 68 kDa in RINm-5F cells. The authors raised the hypothesis that exposure of the normally hidden antigenic determinants may elicit that β cell-specific autoimmune attack although the antigenic epitope is also present in several normally occurring glycolipids.

We have recently described a series of monoclonal autoantibodies derived from prediabetic BB rats. Screening of hybridoma supernatants was carried out on cellular immunoradiometric (Contreas et al. 1986) or ELISA assays using pluripotent rat islet tumor cells, MSL cells (Madsen et al. 1986). A parallel screening was carried out on two related cell lines predominantly expressing the β and δ or α cell phenotype, respectively. Positive clones were then rescreened for reactivity to pancrease sections by indirect immunofluorescence.

Despite the selection criteria for surface binding, we found that some of these monoclonal autoantibodies also reacted to the cytoplasm of subpopulations of islet cells on pancreas sections. This is in contrast to the lack of ICA in BB rat sera (Maclaren et al. 1983). Antibody CA812 selectively stained somatostatin-containing δ cells of the islet, whereas somatostatin cells of the duct did not react (Contreas et al. 1989). Only a fraction of δ cells in the newborn pancreas was labeled (Contreas et al. 1989). Antibody EB52 stained a majority of PP cells, but also a few α cells. Antibody F44 reacted to islet β cells (Fig. 1A), but also to small, scattered groups of exocrine cells (Fig. 1C); the reaction was only observed on frozen sections of rat pancreas and was highly dependent on proper handling of the tissue. Since, when compared with EB52 and CA812, there is increased staining of exocrine tissue, it is likely that the F44 antigen is expressed in all acinar cells, but to a lesser extent. In fact, from the result of immunoblotting of membrane preparations from a variety of rat organs, the F44 antigen of 72 kDa was shown to be widely distributed (Contreas et al. 1988). Antibody EA512 did not stain tissue sections, but revealed a specific binding to two protein bands (M_r 100 and 23 kDa) by immunoblotting, where the high molecular weight band seemed to be endocrine specific (Contreas et al. 1988).

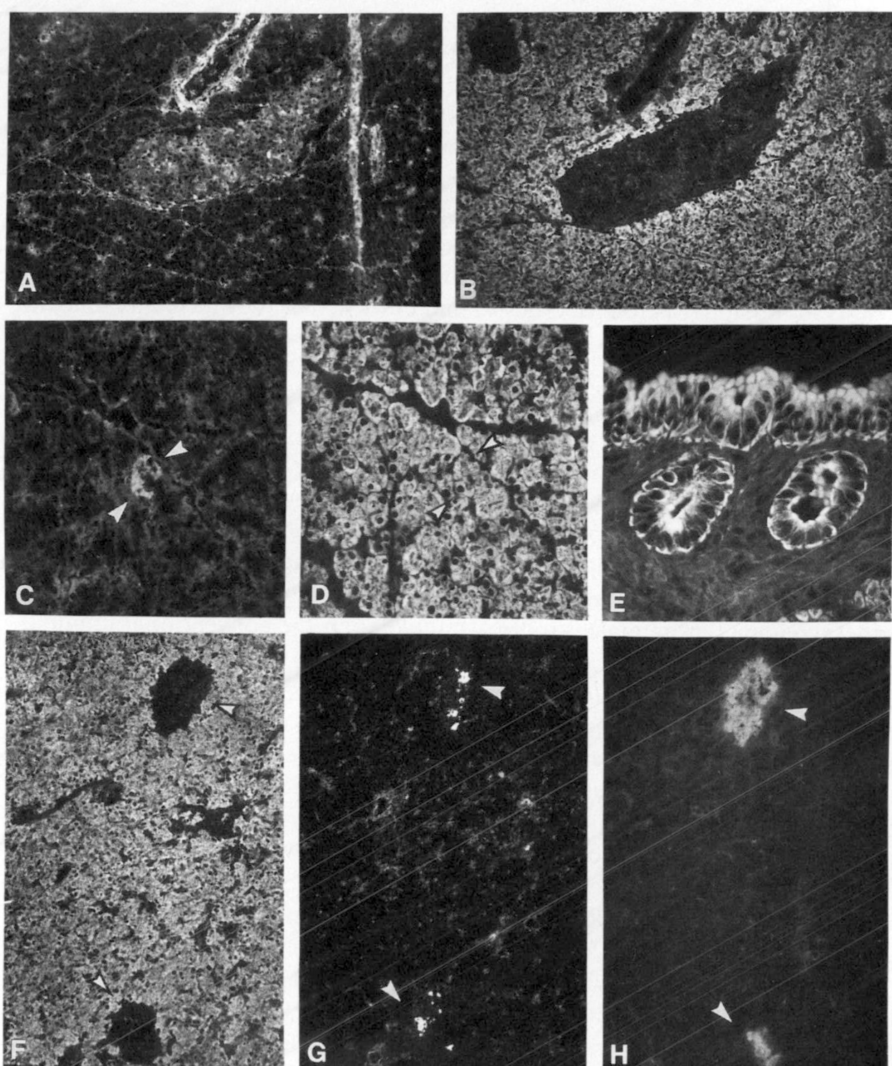

Fig. 1A–H. Antibody staining of sections of rat pancreas by indirect immunofluorescence. **A, B** Serial sections showing islet β cell staining with monoclonal autoantibody F44 (**A**) and acinar cell staining with the panexocrine-reacting H37 monoclonal autoantibody (**B**). **C, D** Serial sections of acinar tissue where few scattered exocrine cells are strongly stained with F44 (**C**). These cells are islet hormone negative and stained by the exocrine acinar cell specific autoantibody, H37, in **D** (*arrow*). **E** The monoclonal autoantibody DA39 stains the entire ductal epithelium of the pancreas, including scattered endocrine cells of the duct. The outer epithelial layer of the entire gastrointestinal tract is also labeled with this antibody (not shown). **F–H** Serial sections of pancreas from a diabetic BB/H rat stained with H37 (**F**) which localizes two unstained islets (*arrow*). The islets contain several CA812 positive islet δ cells (**G**) but the glucagon producing α cell dominates the islets (**H**). The monoclonal glucagon specific antibody Glu-001 (Table 1) was used for staining in **H**. The islet structures were not stained by insulin antibodies or by F44, whereas scattered F44 positive exocrine cells were present (as in **C**, not shown)

Interestingly, antibody H37 (Fig. 1B and 1D) and DA39 stained exocrine acinar cells and duct cells, respectively (Table 3). DA39 stained the entire ductal epithelium (Fig. 1e), including endocrine cells of the duct (CONTREAS et al. 1989).

The involvement of any of these autoantibodies in the pathogenesis of IDDM in the BB rat is not clearly evident since all staining patterns described above are retained in the diabetic pancreas (Fig. 1F, G and H), with the exception of F44 β cell staining. However, according to a recent hypothesis on IDDM pathogenesis where the β cell is not necessarily the target of the initial lesion in the pancreas (NERUP et al. 1987), passive immunization tests must still be carried out with the various monoclonal autoantibodies to find out whether they have any influence on the onset of IDDM in the BB rat.

5 Discussion

Despite the intense efforts of many laboratories, it has not yet been possible to isolate a monoclonal antibody with a documented diabetogenic effect in vivo. The strategy of making monoclonal autoantibodies by fusing lymphocytes from diabetic patients or animals is more attractive than the conventional immunization scheme using isolated islet cell material as antigen. Potential IDDM related autoantibodies are likely to be present in the hybridoma repertoire after a successful high yield fusion, but it should be kept in mind that fusion of lymphocytes, even from healthy individuals, produces a certain frequency of naturally occurring autoantibodies against islet cells (YOON et al. 1984; PRABHAKAR et al. 1984). Such antibodies are often reacting to multiple organs (HASPEL et al. 1983). Therefore, the next question is how to detect and identify an IDDM-relevant (auto)antibody.

The source of target antigen material employed in screening of hybridoma fusions is critical. High yield hybridoma fusions, a prerequisite of ensuring an appropriate spectrum of the (auto)immune repertoire, require very efficient and large scale screening assays. Therefore, islet tumor cells have been used as the most common target cell since they are available in sufficient quantities. We used MSL cells (MADSEN et al. 1986) which are derived from the same original rat insulinoma (CHICK et al. 1977) as the more commonly used RIN-m cells (OIE et al. 1983). The MSL cells possess a remarkable differentiation potential and a particular clone, MSL-G2, has been useful for the study of β cell differentiation in vivo (MADSEN et al. 1988). We have thus derived a β cell tumor line (MSL-G2-IN) where very small sized tumors (< 200 mg) produce hypoglycemia in histocompatible rats.

However, it remains to be shown whether such transformed islet cells in fact express relevant β cell-specific autoantigens. Preliminary data show that the 64-kDa protein is not expressed in MSL-G2-IN tumor cells (S. BAEKKESKOV and O.D. MADSEN, unpublished) and it has not consistently been found in any other source of transformed islet cells. To unambiguously identify the presence of

IDDM-related autoantigen expression by transformed β cells, it will be necessary to produce tumor histocompatible rats carrying the diabetic trait from the BB strain. Such studies are in progress, as are studies on transformed glucagon cells (MSL-G-AN); (MADSEN et al. 1987) which will serve as a unique control to study the selective rejection of β cell tumors.

Acknowledgment. We wish to thank Mrs Bente Völer for expert secretarial assistance in typing this manuscript.

References

Atkinson MA, Maclaren NK (1988) Autoantibodies in non-obese diabetic mice immunoprecipitate 64000 M_r islet antigen. Diabetes 37: 1587–1590

Bækkeskov S, Christie M 1989 (to be published) Characterization of the 64 KD membrane autoantigen in pancreatic β-cells. Current communications in molecular biology. Proceedings of Cold Spring Habour Laboratory Symposium on β-cells. Cold Spring Harbour Laboratory, USA

Bækkeskov S, Nielsen JH, Marner B, Bilde T, Ludvigsson J, Lernmark Å (1982) Autoantibodies in newly diagnosed diabetic children immunoprecipitate specific human pancreatic islet cell proteins. Nature 298: 167–169

Bækkeskov S, Dyrberg T, Lernmark Å (1984) Autoantibodies against an M_r 64 k islet cell protein precede the onset of insulin-dependent diabetes in the BB rat. Science 224: 1348–1350

Bazin H (1982) Production of rat monoclonal antibodies with the LOU rat non-secreting IR983F myeloma cell line. In: Peeters H (ed) Protides of the biological fluids. 29th Colloquium 1981. Pergamon, Oxford, pp 615–618

Boitard C, Bendelac A, Richard MF, Carnaud C, Bach JF (1988) Prevention of diabetes in nonobese diabetic mice by anti-I-A monoclonal antibodies: transfer of protection by splenic T cells Proc Natl Acad Sci USA 85: 9719–9723

Bottazzo GF, Florin-Christensen A, Doniach D (1974) Islet cell antibodies in diabetes mellitus with autoimmune polyendocrine deficiencies. Lancet 2: 1279–1282

Brogren CH, Hirsch F, Wood P, Druet P, Poussier P (1986) Production and characterization of a monoclonal islet cell surface autoantibody from the BB rat. Diabetologia 29: 330–333

Bucchini D, Madsen O, Desbois P, Pictet R, Jami J (1989) B islet cells of pancreas are the site of expression of the human insulin gene in transgenic mice. Exp Cell Res 180: 467–474

Buschard K, Brogren CH, Röpke C, Rygaard J (1988) Antigen expression of the pancreatic beta-cell is dependent on their functional state, as shown by a specific, BB rat monoclonal autoantibody IC2. APMIS 96: 342–346

Buse JB, Powers A, Mori H, Rabizadeh A, Haynes B, Eisenbarth GS (1983) Anti-islet monoclonal autoantibodies from the BB-rat. Diabetes 32: 51A

Charles MA, Suzuki M, Waldeck N, Dodson LE, Slater L, Ono K, Kershnar A, Buckingham B, Golden M (1983) Immune islet killing mechanisms associated with insulin-dependent diabetes: in vitro expression of cellular and antibody-mediated islet cell cytotoxicity in humans. J Immunol 130: 1189–1194

Chick WL, Warren S, Chute RN, Like AA, Lauris V, Kitchen KC (1977) A transplantable insulinoma in the rat. Proc Natl Acad Sci USA 74: 628–632

Colman PG, Nayak RC, Campbell IL, Eisenbarth GS (1988) Binding of cytoplasmic islet cell antibodies is blocked by human pancreatic glycolipid extracts. Diabetes 37: 645–652

Contreas G, Madsen OD, Vissing H, Lernmark Å (1986) A simple assay for the detection of antibodies to endocrine islet cell surface antigens. J Immunol Methods 95: 135–139

Contreas G, Jørgensen JL, Nielsen E, Madsen OD (1988) Characterization by immunoblotting of autoantigens recognized by autoantibodies derived from prediabetic B-rats. In: Schafer-Nielsen C (ed) Electrophoresis '88. Proceedings. Protein Laboratory, University of Copenhagen, pp 432–439

Contreas G, Jørgensen J, Madsen OD (1989) Novel islet, duct and acinar cell markers defined by monoclonal autoantibodies from prediabetic BB rats. Pancreas (in press)

Croce CM, Linnenbach A, Hall W, Steplewski Z, Koprowski H (1980) Production of human hybridomas secreting antibodies to measles virus. Nature 288: 488–489

Dean M, Maker F, McNally JM, Tarn AC, Schwarz G, Gale EAM, Bottazzo GF (1986) Insulin autoantibodies in the pre-diabetic period: correlation with islet cell antibodies and development of diabetes. Diabetologia 29: 339–342

DelPrete GF, Betterle C, Padovan D (1977) Incidence of isletcell autoantibodies in different types of diabetes mellitus. Diabetes 26: 909–915

de St Groth SF, Scheidegger D (1980) Production of monoclonal antibodies: strategy and tactics. J Immunol Methods 35: 1–21

Doberson MJ, Scharff J, Ginsberg-Fellner F, Notkins A (1980) Cytotoxic antibodies to beta cells in the serum of patients with insulin-dependent diabetes mellitus. N Engl J Med 303: 1493–1498

Dyrberg T, Poussier P, Nakhooda AF, Marliss EB, Lernmark Å (1984) Islet cell surface and lymphocyte antibodies often precede the spontaneous diabetes in the BB rat. Diabetologia 26: 159–165

Eisenbarth GS (1987) Genes, generator of diversity, glycoconjugates, and autoimmune β-cell insufficiency in type 1 diabetes. Diabetes 36: 355–364

Eisenbarth GS, Linnenbach A, Jackson R, Scearce R, Croce CM (1982) Human hybridomas secreting anti-islet autoantibodies. Nature 300: 264–267

Eisenbarth GS, Jackson R, Srikanta S, Powers A, Buse J, Mori H (1984) Utilization of monoclonal antibody techniques to study type I (insulin dependent) diabetes mellitus. In: Andreani D, Di Mario U, Federlin KF, Heding LG (eds) Immunology of diabetes. Kimpton Medical, London, pp 143–157

Galfre G, Milstein C, Wright B (1979) Rat x rat hybrid myelomas and a monoclonal anti-Fd portion of mouse IgG. Nature 277: 131–133

Gledhill RM, Mirza IH, Keller U, Leslie RDG, Norman MR, Wilkin TJ (1987) Production of human monoclonal autoantibodies to insulin. Diabetologia 30: 524A

Gray IP, Siddle K, Frank BH, Hales CN (1987) Characterization and use in immunoradiometric assays of monoclonal antibodies directed against human proinsulin. Diabetes 36: 684–688

Grimaldi KA, Hutton JC, Siddle K (1987) Production and characterization of monoclonal antibodies to insulin secretory granule membranes. Biochem J 245: 557–566

Hari J, Yokono K, Yonezawa K, Amano K, Yaso S, Shii K, Imamura Y, Baba S (1986) Immunochemical characterization of antiislet cell surface monoclonal antibody from non-obese diabetic mice. Diabetes 35: 517–522

Haspel MV, Onodera T, Prabhakar BS, McClintock PR, Essani K, Ray UR, Yagihashi S, Notkins AL (1983) Multiple organ-reactive monoclonal autoantibodies. Nature 304: 73–76

Kaplan DR, Colca JR, McDaniel ML (1983) Insulin as a surface marker on isolated cells from rat pancreatic islets. J Cell Biol 97: 453–457

Kearney JF, Radbruch AD, Liezegang B, Rajewsky K (1979) A new mouse myeloma cell line that has lost immunoglobulin expression but permits the construction of antibody-secreting hybrid cell lines. J Immunol 123: 1548–1550

Keilacker H, Dietz H, Witt S, Woltanski KP, Berling R, Ziegler M (1986) Kinetic properties of monoclonal insulin antibodies. Biomed Biochim Acta 45: 1093–1102

Koevary S, Williams D, Williams R, Chick WJ (1985) Passive transfer of diabetes from BB/W to Wistar-Furth rats. J Clin Invest 75: 1904–1907

Köhler G, Milstein C (1975) Continuous cultures of fused cells secreting antibody of predefined specificity. Nature 256: 495–497

Larsson LI, Nielsen JH, Hutton JC, Madsen OD (1989) Pancreatic hormones are expressed on the surfaces of human and rat islet cells through exocytotic sites. Eur J Cell Biol 48: 45–51

Lendrum R, Walker G, Cudworth AG, Theophanides C, Pyke DA, Bloom AJ, Gamble DR (1976) Islet cell antibodies in diabetes mellitus. Lancet 2: 1273–1276

Lernmark Å (1987) Islet cell antibodies. Diabetic Med 4: 285–292

Lernmark Å, Freedman ZR, Hofmann C, Rubenstein AH, Steiner DF, Jackson RL, Winter RJ, Traisman HS (1978) Islet cell surface antibodies in juvenile diabetes mellitus. N Engl J Med 299: 375–380

Lernmark Å, Bækkeskov S, Dyrberg T, Gerling I, Marner B, Papadopoulos G, Svenningsen A, Binder C, Christy M, Nerup J, Mandrup-Poulsen T (1984) Pathogenesis of type 1 diabetes mellitus. In: Labrie F, Proulx L (eds) Endocrinology. Elsevier Science, Amsterdam, pp 92–96

MacCuish AC, Irvine WJ, Baines EW, Duncan LJ (1974) Antibodies to pancreatic islet cells in insulin-dependent diabetics with coexistent autoimmune disease. Lancet 2: 1529–1531

Maclaren NK, Elder ME, Robbins VW, Riley WJ (1983) Autoimmune diathesis and T lymphocyte immunoincompetences in BB rat. Metabolism 32 [Suppl 1]: 92–96

Madsen OD (1987) Proinsulin-specific monoclonal antibodies. Immunocytochemical application as β cell markers and as probes for conversion. Diabetes 36: 1203–1211

Madsen OD, Cohen RM, Fitch FW, Rubenstein AH, Steiner DF (1983a) The production and characterization of monoclonal antibodies specific for human proinsulin using a sensitive microdot assay procedure. Endocrinology 113: 2135–2144

Madsen OD, Carroll RJ, Steiner DF (1983b) Monoclonal antibodies against rat islet cells. Metabolism 32 [Suppl 1]: 165–166

Madsen OD, Frank BH, Steiner DF (1984) Human proinsulin-specific antigenic determinants identified by monoclonal antibodies. Diabetes 33: 1012–1016

Madsen OD, Larsson LI, Rehfeld JF, Schwartz TW, Lernmark Å, Labrecque AD, Steiner DF (1986) Cloned cell lines from a transplantable islet cell tumor are heterogeneous and express cholecystokinin in addition to islet hormones. J Cell Biol 103: 2025–2034

Madsen OD, Rehfeld J, Holst JJ, Kofod H, Hansen B, Lernmark Å (1987) CCK/Glucagon expression selectively follows an anorectic tumor phenotype formed from pluripotent transformed islet cells. J Steroid Biochem 28 [Suppl]: 128S

Madsen OD, Andersen LC, Michelsen B, Owerbach D, Larsson LI, Lernmark Å, Steiner DF (1988) Tissue-specific expression of transfected human insulin genes in pluripotent clonal rat insulinoma lines induced during passage in vivo. Proc Natl Acad Sci USA 85: 6652–6656

Makino S, Kunimoto R, Muraoka Y, Mizushima Y, Katagiri K, Tochino Y (1980) Breeding of a non-obese diabetic strain of mice. Exp Animals 29: 1–13

Marliss EB (1983) Workshop on the spontaneously diabetic BB rat. Metabolism 32 [Suppl 1]: 1–166

Maruyama T, Takei I, Yanagawa T, Takahashi T, Asaba Y, Kataoka K, Ishii T (1988) Insulin autoantibodies in non-obese diabetic (NOD) mice and streptozotocin-induced diabetic mice. Diabetes Res 7: 93–96

Nayak RC, Omar MAK, Rabizadeh A, Srikanta S, Eisenbarth GS (1985) "Cytoplasmic" islet cell antibodies: evidence that the target antigen is a sialoglycoconjugate. Diabetes 34: 617–619

Nerup J, Mandrup-Poulsen T, Mølvig J (1987) The HLA-IDDM association: implications for etiology and pathogenesis of IDDM. Diabetes Metab Rev 3: 779–802

Oie HK, Gazdar AF, Minna JD, Weir G, Baylin SB (1983) Clonal analysis of insulin and somatostatin secretion and *L*-dopa decarboxylase expression by a rat islet cell tumor. Endocrinology 112: 1070–1075

Orci L, Ravazzola M, Amherdt M, Madsen O, Vassalli JD, Perrelet A (1985) Direct identification of prohormone conversion site in insulin-secreting cells. Cell 42: 671–681

Orci L, Ravazzola M, Amherdt M, Madsen O, Perrelet A, Vassalli JD, Anderson RGW (1986) Conversion of proinsulin to insulin occurs coordinately with acidification of maturing secretory vesicles. J Cell Biol 103: 2273–2281

Orci L, Ravazzolla M, Amherdt M, Perrelet A, Powell SK, Quinn DL, Moore HPH (1987a) The trans-most cisternae of the Golgi complex: a compartment for sorting of secretory and plasma membrane proteins. Cell 51: 1039–1051

Orci L, Ravazzola M, Storch MJ, Anderson RGW, Vassalli JD, Perrelet A (1987b) Proteolytic maturation of insulin is a post-Golgi event which occurs in acidifying clathrin-coated secretory vesicles. Cell 49: 865–868

Palmer JP, Asplin CM, Clemons P, Lyen K, Tatpati O, Raghu PK, Paquette TL (1983) Insulin antibodies in insulin-dependent diabetics before insulin treatment. Science 222: 1337–1339

Poussier P, Dayer-Métroz MD (1988) Monoclonal islet cell antibodies. In: Shafrir E, Renold AE (eds) Frontiers in diabetes research. Lessons from animal diabetes II John Libbey, London, pp 46–51

Poussier P, Legendre C, Wood P, Guttmann RD, Brogren C-H (1986) Identification of a common epitope on the surface of rat islet cells and thymic T lymphocytes using monoclonal antibody (MAB) produced from the BB-rat. Diabetes 35 [Suppl] 1: 25A

Prabhakar BS, Saegusa J, Onodera T, Notkins AL (1984) Lymphocytes capable of making monoclonal autoantibodies that react with multiple organs are a common feature of the normal B cell repertoire. J Immunol 133: 2815–2817

Rabinovitch A, Mackay P, Ludvigsson J, Lernmark Å (1984) A prospective analysis of islet cell cytotoxic antibodies in insulin-dependent diabetic children: transient effects of plasmapheresis. Diabetes 33: 224–228

Sai P, Maurel C, Kremer M, Barriere P (1984) Monoclonal anti-islet cell autoantibodies from C_{57}BLKsJ db/db diabetic mice. Hybridoma 3: 131–139

Schatz DA, Barrett DJ, Maclaren NK, Riley WJ (1988) Polyclonal nature of islet cell antibodies in insulin dependent diabetes. Autoimmunity 1: 45–50

Schroer JA, Bender T, Feldmann RJ, Kim KJ (1983) Mapping epitopes on the insulin molecule using monoclonal antibodies. Eur J Immunol 14: 693–700

Schulman M, Wilde CD, Köhler G (1978) A better cell line for making hybridomas secreting specific antibodies. Nature 276: 269–270

Storch MJ, Petersen KG, Licht T, Kerp L (1985) Recognition of human insulin and proinsulin by monoclonal antibodies. Diabetes 34: 808–811

Srikanta S, Eisenbarth GS (1986) Islet cell antigens. Initial studies of their biology and function. Mol Biol Med 3: 113–127

Takei I, Maruyama T, Taniyama M, Kataoka K (1986) Humoral immunity in the NOD mouse. In: Tarui S, Tochino Y, Nonaka K (eds) Insulitis and type 1 diabetes. Lessons from the NOD mouse. Academic Press, Tokyo, pp 101–110

Teng NNH, Lam KS, Riera FC, Kaplan HS (1983) Construction and testing of mouse–human heteromyelomas for human monoclonal antibody production. Proc Natl Acad Sci USA 80: 7308–7312

Uchigata Y, Spitalnik SL, Tachiwaki O, Salata KF, Notkins AL (1987) Pancreatic islet cell surface glycoproteins containing Galβ1-4GlcNAc-R identified by a cototoxic monoclonal auto-antibody. J Exp Med 165: 124–139

Vardi P, Dibella EE, Pasquarello TJ, Srikanta S (1987) Islet cell autoantibodies: pathobiology and clinical applications. Diabetes Care 10: 645–656

Wilkin T, Hoskins PJ, Armitage M, Rodier M, Casey C, Diaz JL, Pyke DA, Lesley RDG (1985) Value of insulin autoantibodies as serum markers for insulin dependent diabetes mellitus. Lancet 1: 480–481

Wilkin T, Kiesel U, Diaz JL, Burkart V, Korb H (1986) Auto-antibodies to insulin as serum markers for autoimmune insulitis. Diabetes Res 3: 173–174

Witt S, Hehmke B, Dietz H, Ziegler B, Hildmann W, Ziegler M (1985) Complement-dependent cytotoxicity of monoclonal antibodies against islet cells. Biomed Biochim Acta 44: 117–121

Witt VS, Dietz H, Ziegler B, Keilacker H, Ziegler M (1988) Erzeugung und Anwendung monoklonaler Glucagon-und Insulinantikörper-Reduktion des Pankreasinsulins bei Ratten durch Behandlung mit komplettem Freundschen Adjuvans. Acta Histochem [Suppl] 35: 217–223

Yokono K, Shii K, Hari J, Yaso S, Imamura Y, Ejiri K, Ishihara K, Fujii S, Kazumi T, Taniguchi H, Baba S (1984) Production of monoclonal antibodies to islet cell surface antigens using hybridization of spleen lymphocytes from non-obese diabetic mice. Diabetologia 26: 379–385

Yokono K, Amano K, Suenaga K, Hari J, Shii K, Yaso S, Yonezawa K, Imamura Y, Baba S (1986) Effect of antiserum to monoclonal anti-islet cell surface antibody on pancreatic insulitis in non-obese diabetic mice. Diab Res Clin Pract 1: 315–321

Yoon JW, Shin SY, Bachurski CJ (1984) Hybridomas from lymphocytes of normal mice produce monoclonal autoantibodies. Lancet 2: 641

Ziegler M, Ziegler B, Hehmke B (1984) Severe hyperglycemia caused by autoimmunization to beta cells in rat. Diabetologia 27: 163–165

Ziegler M, Teneberg S, Witt S, Ziegler B, Hehmke B, Kohnert KD, Egeberg J, Karlsson KA, Lernmark Å (1988) Islet β-cytotoxic monoclonal antibody against glycolipids in experimental diabetes induced by low dose streptozotocin and Freund's adjuvant. J Immunol 140: 4144–4150

The Genetics of Insulin-Dependent Diabetes in the BB Rat

W. KASTERN[1], F. LANG[1], and I. KRYSPIN-SØRENSEN[2]

1 Introduction

1.1 Human IDDM

The susceptibility towards the development of type 1 or insulin-dependent diabetes mellitus (IDDM) in humans is inherited in a complex and, as yet, unclear fashion. At least one genetic component is linked to the class II region of the major histocompatibility complex (MHC), but this component appears to be insufficient in determining susceptibility towards the disease. The identification of a gene or combination of genes which leads to the development of the disease has been hampered by the diverse genetic background of the human population, possible heterogeneity within the disease itself, and the low penetrance of the gene(s) involved.

1.2 The Genetics of Diabetes in the NOD Mouse

The availability of two excellent animal models for type 1 diabetes promises to lead to a better understanding of genetic mechanisms which can cause the autoimmune destruction of the beta cells in the pancreatic islets of Langerhans. In the nonobese diabetic (NOD) mouse, at least three recessive genes are involved (see review by HANAFUSA and TARUI, this volume). As in human IDDM, one of the disease genes is linked to the mouse MHC on chromosome 17 (HATTORI et al. 1986). Outcross of the NOD to a related inbred strain followed by backcross of the F_1 progeny to the NOD revealed that there were at least two additional genes necessary for diabetes (PROCHAZKA et al. 1987). The first of these genes was mapped to chromosome 9 within a 25 centimorgan (cM) region between the centromere and the Alp-1 locus (PROCHAZKA et al. 1987). The second of these two

[1] University of Florida College of Medicine, Department of Pathology, Box J-275, JHMHC, Gainesville, FL 32610, USA
[2] Danish National Food Agency, DK-2860 Soborg, Denmark

Current Topics in Microbiology and Immunology, Vol. 156

genes has not, as yet, been mapped (Prochazka et al. 1987; Leiter and Prochazka 1988). While these three genes which lead to diabetes in the NOD mouse have not been identified, it is clear that the inheritance of diabetes is under polygenic control in this model.

2 The Genetics of Diabetes in the BB Rat

2.1 The MHC Component of BB Rat Diabetes

The inheritance of IDDM in the BB rat also involves several genes. As in human and NOD mouse diabetes, there is a requirement for a specific MHC haplotype ($RT1^u$) in the BB rat (Colle et al. 1981). The MHC component of diabetes in the BB rat is a dominant one since heterozygotes for $RT1^u$ could also develop the disease (Guttmann et al. 1983; Colle et al. 1983; Jackson et al. 1984). This component of the disease is an example of a normal allele which is necessary for the susceptibility to the disease since the $RT1^u$ could be inherited from other strains unrelated to the BB and still permit the disease to occur (Colle et al. 1986). In this study, healthy PVG.r8 rats ($RT1.A^aB^uD^u$) were crossed with diabetic BB hooded rats ($RT1.A^uB^uD^u$). In the F_2 generation, two out of eight diabetic animals were typed as homozygous for the PVG.r8 MHC, indicating that the PVG alleles at the class II MHC loci were able to permit the development of diabetes in those rats (Colle et al. 1986). In this regard, the MHC-linked diabetes susceptibility gene may be considered a normal allele since none of the several rat strains that have this allele (e.g., Wistar Furth) show any noticeable defects. Recently, the nucleotide sequence of the messenger RNAs that code for the class II beta chains were shown to be identical in the diabetes-prone BB, the diabetes-resistant BB, and Wistar Furth rats (Holowachuk and Greer 1989). Thus, the MHC requirement for diabetes in the rat is only for a "u" allele and not any particular, or mutant, "u" allele.

This ability to utilize any "u" allele indicated that the mutations responsible for the development of diabetes in the BB rat were not located within the MHC, and that the MHC haplotype was merely permissive for the development of the disease when inherited with the proper combination of other susceptibility genes. While there are no mutations within the MHC of the BB rat, it is unclear what role these antigens play in the development of the disease. Recent evidence has indicated that the pancreatic islets of prediabetic BB rats have an increased expression of class I MHC antigens (Ono et al. 1988). This expression appeared to be a severalfold increase over the expression in islets of non-diabetes-prone rats as seen by RNA dot blot hybridization. Since the regulation of class I expression could be controlled by trans-acting factors expressed at other genetic loci, these observations remain consistent with the lack of linkage between a mutant MHC gene and diabetes in the rat.

2.2 Lymphopenia

Estimates of the number of other genes involved in the pathogenesis of IDDM in the BB rat have varied, depending on the strain of rat used to perform the outcross with. A gene which seems to be universally necessary is that responsible for the severe T cell lymphopenia observed in peripheral blood and lymphoid tissues of the diabetic rats (JACKSON et al. 1984; POUSSIER et al. 1982). The gene for this trait has been shown to be necessary for the development of IDDM in the BB rat because the disease was very tightly linked to lymphopenia (GUTTMANN et al. 1983; JACKSON et al. 1984). Since the lymphopenia gene is known to be inherited as an autosomal recessive with complete penetrance (JACKSON et al. 1984), one can consider this gene as the mutant "diabetes gene." In this regard, the lymphopenia gene was a spontaneously arising trait that had not been observed previously; it was an allele that was definitely not normal, and only the allele from the BB rat could lead to the disease.

Recently, results from two laboratories have demonstrated that lymphopenia was perhaps not an absolute requirement for IDDM in the BB rat (LIKE et al. 1986; HEROLD et al. 1989; GUBERSKI et al. 1989). In one case, several diabetic animals that had normal percentages of T cell subsets were discovered in a line of diabetes-resistant BB rats (LIKE et al. 1986). Crosses of these nonlymphopenic diabetic (NLD) animals with lymphopenic diabetic BB rat resulted in 5 NLD animals out of 475 (1%) in the F_2 generation (GUBERSKI et al. 1989). In the other case, a cross between a diabetic animal and an animal from a BB diabetes-resistant line resulted in a number of F_2 animals that were diabetic without lymphopenia (HEROLD et al. 1989). However, several aspects of the diabetes suffered by these animals indicated that the IDDM was atypical and perhaps different from the disorder usually seen in the BB rat. The age at onset of nonlymphopenic diabetes (usually less than 70 days of age) was earlier than the 90–100 days normally seen in the BB rat (HEROLD et al. 1989; GUBERSKI et al. 1989). A cross between NLD and lymphopenic diabetic BB rats did not produce diabetic animals in the F_1 generation, indicative that different genes were involved in the pathogenesis of the two forms of diabetes (GUBERSKI et al. 1989). Similarly, a cross between two NLD animals resulted in 0/23 diabetics in the F_1 generation (GUBERSKI et al. 1989). Moreover, the appearance of nonlymphopenic diabetes was sudden and in a line in which diabetes had not been detected in 9–12 generations (LIKE et al. 1986). Likewise, the appearance of NLD animals in the F_2 generation of a cross between diabetes-resistant and diabetic BB rats was also sudden and not previously seen in similar crosses (HEROLD et al. 1989). A single NLD animal was observed out of 11 animals in the F_1 generation of a cross between a BB and a Buffalo rat (GUTTMANN et al. 1983). This was surprising because this has been the only published observation of an F_1 diabetic in an outcross of the BB, an indication of dominant genes in the absence of recessives. These aspects of nonlymphopenic diabetes together with the inability to demonstrate Mendelian inheritance of the trait suggest a possible environmental explanation for the development of this form of IDDM in the BB rat.

2.3 Other Genes

2.3.1 The Problem of Assessing the Total Number of Genes Involved

An understanding of the genes involved in the pathogenesis of a multigenic disorder such as diabetes is complicated by the tendency to refer to these genes as "diabetes genes" or "diabetogenic genes." These terms have the connotations that each of them carry a specific mutation or defect which causes the disease. Rather than needing to account for the simultaneous occurrence of at least two or three different mutations in a parental animal line, resulting in the sudden appearance of the disease, it is more likely that a single mutation occurred in one gene. This mutation would probably not have been noticed except for its chance occurrence against a background of genetic conditions which were permissive for the development of the disease. In a genetic analysis of the inheritance of the disease, all of the genes would be classified as diabetogenic genes when, in reality, they were probably normal alleles that were present in the population. These genes are not to be considered diabetogenic in the sense that they actually cause the disease. Rather, they merely provide the proper environment for the actual mutant gene to cause the disease.

The purpose of such a distinction is important for the study of the inheritance of the disease since different populations (whether they are inbred animals or humans) will have different frequencies of the normal alleles which provide the susceptibility to the disease. These differences lead to varying estimates of the frequency of the disease as well as seemingly contradictory observations about the number of genes necessary for the disease. Regardless of whether a gene is a mutant or a normal allele, it is important to study its involvement in the pathogenesis of a disease because a full understanding of all the factors which cause the disease is necessary. With regard to inbred animal models, the combination of genes necessary for a disease is usually detected through multiple outcrosses of the afflicted animal strain with other strains. This is because only a single outcross with a particular strain may hide the need for a certain gene since the disease allele may be present in both strains. Through several outcrosses, one can lessen the probability of missing the involvement of any of the necessary genes.

2.3.2 Results of Outcrossing the BB Rat with Other Strains

The inheritance of IDDM in the BB rat is confusing and is a good example of how the number of genes involved can vary with the strain of rat used for the outcross. In crosses between the diabetes-prone and diabetes-resistant lines of inbred BB rat, the incidence of diabetes is 20%–25% in the F_2 generation, consistent with a single recessive gene for diabetes (Bjørck et al. 1986; Kryspin-Sørensen et al. 1986; Herold et al. 1989; Guberski et al. 1989). However, in crosses between the diabetes-prone BB and other strains of rats, the incidence of diabetes in the F_2 generation is much lower and suggests that more genes must be involved (Table 1).

Table 1. Incidence of diabetes in the F_2 generations of outcrosses of the BB rat with other strains

Outcross strain	MHC haplotype	F_2 incidence of IDDM (%)	Reference
BB-DR	$RT1^u$	15/78 (19)	KRYSPIN-SØRENSEN et al. 1986
BB-DR	$RT1^u$	26/86 (30)	HEROLD et al. 1989
BB-DR	$RT1^u$	107/475 (22.5)	GUBERSKI et al. 1989
Buffalo	$RT1^b$	5/101 (5.0)	GUTTMANN et al. 1983
Lewis	$RT1^l$	4/128 (3.1)	COLLE et al. 1983
Wistar Furth	$RT1^u$	6/251 (2.4)	JACKSON et al. 1984
Brown Norway	$RT1^n$	18/949 (1.9)	JACKSON et al. 1984
Lewis	$RT1^l$	8/351 (2.3)	JACKSON et al. 1984
Long Evans	$RT1^{uv}$	6/89 (7.0)	MARKHOLST and KASTERN, unpublished
Long Evans	$RT1^{uv}$	15/207 (7.5)	LANG and KASTERN 1989
NEDH	$RT1^g$	1/25 (4.0)	MARKHOLST, unpublished
Wistar Furth	$RT1^u$	1/93 (1.0)	MARKHOLST, unpublished

This indicates that the diabetes-prone BB and its sister line, the diabetes-resistant BB, share all but one recessive allele necessary for the development of IDDM. In an effort to reconcile these differences and as an approach towards the eventual identification of all genes involved, we will discuss the various genetic crosses that have been published involving the BB rat.

As already stated, crosses between the diabetes-prone and diabetes-resistant lines of the BB rat have generally resulted in an incidence of diabetes in the F_2 generation of 20%–25%. There was also an incidence of lymphopenia at 25% with all diabetics being lymphopenic (KRYSPIN-SØRENSEN et al. 1986; HEROLD et al. 1989). From this, one can conclude that the single recessive gene involved in this cross was the lymphopenia gene. The few animals which were lymphopenic, but not diabetic, were probably attributable to a lower penetrance of other genes necessary for the development of IDDM since the lymphopenia gene is known to be fully penetrant (HEROLD et al. 1989; GUBERSKI et al. 1989; LANG and KASTERN 1989). Another trait which seemed to segregate with diabetes in this cross was the absence of a high molecular weight serum protein that bound β_2-microglobulin (BJØRCK et al. 1986). It is unknown what the role of this complex was, but it was present in all lymphopenic animals and was probably result of the lymphopenia rather than the diabetes.

Much more information about the inheritance of diabetes can be derived from outcrosses of the diabetes-resistant BB rat with other unrelated strains, and a number of these have been performed. In a cross between noninbred BB rats and Buffalo (RTI^b) rats, there was a 5% incidence of diabetes in the F_2 generation (GUTTMANN et al. 1983). In this cross, there appeared to be three genetic components of IDDM: (1) the MHC haplotype was at least heterozygous for the $RT1^u$, (2) all diabetics were lymphopenics, and (3) there appeared to be a gene for pancreatic lymphocytic infiltration necessary for IDDM (GUTTMANN et al. 1983). The 5% incidence in the F_2 animals indicated that more than one gene was necessary for diabetes. This would include a recessive for lymphopenia and a dominant for the MHC component; however, since there was high mortality in both the F_1 and F_2 generations, further conclusions about gene number and dominance or recessiveness was unwarranted.

In a cross between noninbred BB rats with the Lewis (RT1l) strain, there was a 3.1% (4/128) incidence of IDDM in the F_2 generation, again indicative of more than one recessive gene (COLLE et al. 1983). Once again the MHC component was dominant and all diabetics were lymphopenic, but an additional component may have been a gene which was responsible for pancreatic lymphocytic infiltration (PLI). This gene appeared to be inherited in a dominant fahsion with incomplete penetrance, although determination of its phenotype was difficult. The low incidence (3.1%) of IDDM in this cross can be explained either by one recessive (lymphopenia) and two dominants (MHC and PLI) genes with low penetrance or by the involvement of additional dominant genes. Since the MHC and lymphopenia are fully penetrant, the low penetrance must be attributable to the PLI gene, but this does not preclude the inculsion of additional genes into the model.

A thorough study of the inheritance of IDDM in the rat has been described in crosses between the BB-DP and Wistar Furth ($RT1^u$), Brown Norway ($RT1^n$), and Lewis ($RT1^l$; JACKSON et al. 1984). Outcross of the noninbred BB diabetes-prone animals with these three strains resulted in no F_1 diabetics. An intercross of the F_1 animals resulted in a 1.9% (18/949) and 2.3% (8/351) incidence of diabetes in the F_2 generations involving Brown Norway (BN) and Lewis, respectively. Interestingly, the cross involving the Wistar Furth strain, which was also $RT1^u$ and therefore would be expected to satisfy at least that requirement for IDDM, yielded only a 2.4% (6/251) incidence of IDDM in the F_2 animals. Since there was no difference in sequence of the $RT1^u$ class II molecules between DP-BB and Wistar Furth (HOLOWACHUK and GREER 1989), and since $RT1^u$ from other strains was sufficient for the development of IDDM (COLLE et al. 1986), this low incidence would indicate that other genes were involved in the cross between BB-DP and Wistar Furth. An incidence as low as 2.4% could be explained by the single recessive for lymphopenia plus at least one additional recessive and one dominant or multiple dominant genes. Similarly, the crosses which involved BN and Lewis required the lymphopenia (recessive) and MHC (dominant) components plus at least one additional recessive or two dominant genes to explain incidences as low as 1.9% and 2.3% in the F_2 generation.

While the MHC component and the recessive lymphopenia genes have been a consistent requirement for the development of diabetes in the F_2 animals of outcross/intercross breeding programs, it is apparent that the number of other "background" genes which are necessary for IDDM varied from strain to strain. One strain which seemed to give a particularly high incidence of diabetes in an outcross with inbred BB diabetes-prone rats was Long Evans ($RT1^{uv}$), (LANG and KASTERN 1989). In an outcross which we performed between the diabetes-prone BB and Long Evans rats, there was no diabetes in the F_1 animals, but the F_2 generation showed 7.5% incidence of the disease. This fits neither a single recessive (25% incidence of diabetes expected) nor a double recessive (6.25% incidence expected) gene model for the inheritance of the disease. One can construct models which include various combinations of dominant and recessive genes to account for these observations, and further studies concerning this inheritance are in progress. The important consideration is that the higher incidence of diabetes in the F_2 generation of this outcross was due to the fact that one or more of the genes involved are present in the Long Evans animals as normal alleles. A clue in this regard may lie in the MHC haplotype of the Long Evans strain. This haplotype is designated $RT1^{uv}$ ($u^{variant}$) since it resembles the 'u' haplotype in most regards except that it differs at RT1.C loci (Stock and Gunther 1979; Wonigeit et al. 1979). Perhaps the genes that need to be 'u' for the pathogenesis of IDDM are similar enough to the authentic 'u' haplotype so as to be sufficient in this cross. If so, valuable clues as to the identity of these MHC-linked genes can be found from studies which are currently underway in our laboratory.

3 Location of the Diabetes Susceptibility Genes

3.1 Assessment of the Difficulty of Mapping the Genes

The discussion above makes clear the fact that the inheritance of IDDM in the BB rat is complicated and involves a multigenic process. Conventional genetic techniques for mapping the genes are inappropriate for a number of reasons. Since the disease is multigenic, and since only the correct complement of alleles will lead to the disease, it is difficult to follow the individual traits through a pedigree. Indeed, of the genes involved, the only one which could be detected independently of the others would be the lymphopenia gene which is easily detected in the homozygous state. Thus, this would be the only gene which could be transferred to another background for independent analysis. The remainder of the genes must all be studied in the few animals that eventually develop IDDM.

Another difficulty in mapping the diabetes genes in the rat is the lack of a bank of genetic markers with which to study linkage in the rat genome. Few genes, or loci, have actually been assigned to specific rat chromosomes, and, thus far, only 11 linkage groups have been determined (O'Brien 1987). Clearly, most of the rat genome which consits of 21 chromosomes has not yet been mapped with conventional genetic markers. This is compounded by the fact that the various inbred strains of laboratory rat tend to be identical for the various alleles of the known isoenzymes (Bender et al. 1984). This complicates genetic linkage studies since few of the isozyme markers will be informative in any outcross. Any utilization of classical genetic markers will therefore need to involve outcrosses with many strains of rats so as to be able to screen as many loci as possible.

3.2 Detection of Linkage with Polymorphic DNA Restriction Fragments

One means of overcoming the lack of informative genetic markers would be to utilize polymorphic DNA fragments which have been generated by restriction enzymes (see reviews by Botstein et al. 1980; Davies 1981; White 1984). A restriction fragment length polymorphism (RFLP) is the change in length of any DNA fragment due to the insertion or deletion of DNA sequence within a length of DNA, or the alteration of restriction enzyme recognition site by point mutagenesis such that a site is added or deleted. The types of mutation which generate RFLPs frequently appear outside of a protein coding region. Since these noncoding regions do not have the high degree of selective pressure which is inherent in a coding region, RFLPs appear much more frequently than the kinds of mutations which would alter the electrophoretic mobility of an isoenzyme. The use of RFLP analysis has proven to be quite powerful in genetic mapping, and a number of diseases have been mapped by these methods when more conventional genetic methods failed. Some examples of diseases which have been mapped by the use of random markers are cystic fibrosis (Knowlton et al. 1985), Huntington's disease (Gilliam et al. 1987), Duchenne muscular dystrophy (Murray et al. 1982), and bilateral acoustic neurofibromatosis (Rouleau et al. 1987).

The easiest mode of linking polymorphic DNA fragments to a disease would be if a cloned gene known to be involved in the disease could be used as a probe of Southern blots. In this manner one could ignore the remainder of the genome and test the inheritance of RFLPs within that gene for linkage to the disease. However, most disease proceed by unknown mechanisms with no clue to the gene(s) responsible. Thus, one does not have the use of cloned genes responsible for these diseases. The task of establishing linkage becomes much more formidable in this case. One could begin testing methodically all cloned genes in the hope that one may show linkage to the disease. However, this would be tedious and time-consuming due to the amount of work needed to test a single gene. Moreover, the size of the mammalian genome (i.e., 3×10^9 base pairs or 3000 centimorgans) means that one would need at least 150 markers equally spaced 20 centimorgans (cM) apart in the genome in order to test every region for linkage (Botstein et al. 1980). Since 150 DNA markers conveniently spaced 20 cM apart are not available, many more markers would need to be screened for linkage. Clearly, this is a formidable undertaking beyond the resources of any laboratory or group of laboratories, and a more practical approach to the mapping of the diabetes genes is necessary.

3.3 The Use of Repetitive DNA Sequences to Detect Multiple RFLPs

Rather than testing single genes for RFLPs and then testing these for linkage to a trait, much time and effort could be saved if multiple loci could be screened simultaneously. The solution lies not in using single-copy DNA sequences as probes for RFLPs, but rather to use repetitive DNA sequences. These sequences are stretches of DNA, either long or short, which are repeated multiple times in the genome. There are three classes of repetitive sequences as defined by the frequency with which they are repeated in the genome (Table 2); (see reviews by Jelinek and Schmid 1982; Deininger and Daniels 1986). The highly repetitive are repeated millions of times in the genome and are typified by the tandem (clustered) repeats in centromeric DNA. The middle repetitive sequences are repeated over 100000 times/haploid genome. The best-known example of these sequences are the human Alu family of repeated sequences which are repeated approximately 500000 times (see review by Schmid and Jelinek 1982). The moderately repetitive DNA sequences are repeated from 50 to 3000 times per haploid genome, and , finally, the single copy sequences are what we usually think of as genes (Table 2).

3.3.1 The Usefulness of Interspersed, Moderately Repetitive DNA Sequences

The class of repetitive DNA which we are interested in using as probes in linkage studies in the rat are the moderately repetitive sequences. These sequences tend to be interspersed throughout the genome of the rat so that the same sequence appears on several chromosomes and in several different regions (Pearson et al. 1978). The moderately repetitive sequences do not code for proteins, so there is not the strong selective pressure against mutation as with single-copy genes. This, and the fact that they change rapidly due to unequal crossing over, means that they are prone to a high frequency of change or hypervariability (Wyman and White 1980; Jeffreys et al. 1985). Although they do not themselves code for protein, they seem to be located near protein coding regions in the genome and, as such, may play a regulatory role (Britten and Davidson 1969, 1971). Their use as a probe insures the screening of regions of the genome where genes are located. Since they are only repeated a few times (i.e., 50–3000 times/haploid genome), and since many of these repeats are tandem, or clustered, so that several will appear on a single restriction fragment, the banding pattern which they detect on Southern blots is simple enough to analyze as opposed to the smear of hybridizing material which one would see with a highly repetitive DNA probe.

Table 2. Repetitive sequence distribution in rat genomic DNA (from Pearson et al. 1978)

Component	Fraction of genome	Repeats/ haploid genome	Number/genome
1	0.02	> 100000	
2	0.21	3000	50
3	0.10	12.5	350
4	0.67	1	531000

All of these qualities make some of these repetitive sequences, also called minisatellites, very useful in the screening for RFLPs (JEFFREYS et al. 1985; JEFFREYS et al. 1986). In one case, a hypervariable minisatellite sequence proved so useful that it was successfully used for identity verification in an immigration test case (JEFFREYS et al. 1985b), for determination of twin zygosity at birth (HILL and JEFFREYS 1985), and for identification in a forensic case (GILL et al. 1985). Thus, the use of hypervariable repetitive DNA sequences will find a multitude of application in addition to genetic mapping.

3.3.2 Development and Testing of Moderately Repetitive DNA Probes in the RAT

We have developed a number of DNA probes that are repeated throughout the rat genome, by shearing rat DNA to a small size (i.e., 300 base pairs), denaturing it to single-stranded DNA, and allowing it to re-anneal under conditions where only the highly repeated DNA sequences would anneal. This highly repetitive DNA was removed, and the remaining DNA which contained moderately repetitive and single copy sequences was allowed to re-anneal. This time, the reaction was terminated after the moderately repetitive sequences had enough time to anneal. These sequences were then separated, their uneven ends filled in with DNA polymerase (Klenow fragment), ligated to EcoR1 linkers, and cloned into the plasmid, pUC18. By cloning in this manner, we were able to isolate several hundred moderately repetitive DNA sequences from the rat genome (W. KASTERN and I. KRYSPIN-SØRENSEN, unpublished).

Each cloned rat repetitive sequence was tested for a number of parameters which were necessary for them to be useful for screening multiple, unlinked loci in the rat genome. First, it was necessary to determine whether the probe was indeed the member of a moderately repetitive DNA family. For this, portions of genomic DNA from each rat were digested with 1 of a bank of 11 enzymes. The digested DNAs were subjected to electrophoresis on agarose gels to separate the fragments on the basis of size. After transferring the banding pattern from the agarose gels to nylon filters, the radioactively labeled cloned repetitive sequences was used to hybridize to the blotted filter. An example of a Southern blot of rat DNA probed with such a moderately repetitive DNA sequence (Fig. 1b) demonstrates that approximately 20–30 bands can be detected. A comparison is made with the same blot probed with a highly repetitive sequence which detects countless bands at all sizes resulting in a smear (Fig. 1a) and a single-copy sequence which detects only two bands on the blot (Fig. 1c). One can see that the most information can be obtained from the moderately repetitive probe.

The second criterion for selecting a useful probe was that it detect on Southern blots restriction fragments that were polymorphic between various rat strains. This was tested by comparing the patterns obtained when genomic DNAs from different inbred strains were probed with each repetitive probe. An example of this type of hypervariability is a comparison of the diabetes-prone BB/H line with Long Evans rats (Fig. 1d, e). Most of the bands were identical, but several

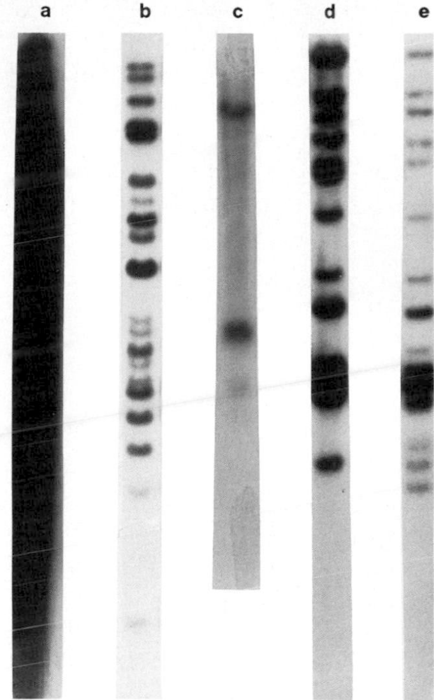

Fig. 1a–e. Repetitive sequences used as probes of Southern blots of rat DNA. To illustrate the banding patterns seen upon probing Southern blots with each of the three families of repetitive sequences as described in the text, ^{32}P-labeled DNA was used to hybridize to DNA blotted to nylon filters. The probes of each lane are **a** highly repetitive DNA sequence, **b** cloned moderately repetitive rat DNA sequence, **c** cloned rat insulin cDNA (represents a single-copy sequence), **d** cloned probe, 4a22a, hybridized with BB rat DNA, and **e** cloned probe, 4a22a, hybridized with Long Evans rat DNA

were noticeably different between the two strains. Each of these polymorphic bands was a potential genetic marker for the disease.

That the repetitive sequences detected by the moderately repetitive DNA probe are interspersed randomly throughout the genome was tested by following the inheritance of each in a pedigree of a cross between the BB/H and Long Evans strains. While some were found to be linked genetically to others, it was clear that the majority of RFLPs segregated from each other. Thus, this probe was able to detect multiple unlinked loci in the rat genome, thereby making the task of screening the entire rat genome much simpler. Using this method, we have isolated three probes which will prove quite useful in our studies. Of these probes 2 (named 4a22a and 37a) detect approximately 50 loci each, and RFLPs have been demonstrated with at least 8 of the tested restriction enzymes. The other is similar to a human repetitive DNA sequence, known as a minisatellite (Jeffreys et al. 1985a), which detects between 50 and 100 (depending on hybridization conditions) unlinked loci in the rat genome.

3.3.3 Initial Screening for Linkage of RFLPs with Diabetes

In initial studies, one of the probes was used to screen the F_2 generation of a cross between the diabetes-prone BB and the Long Evans strain. The restriction enzyme, MspI, was used to digest DNA samples from F_2 individuals, followed by

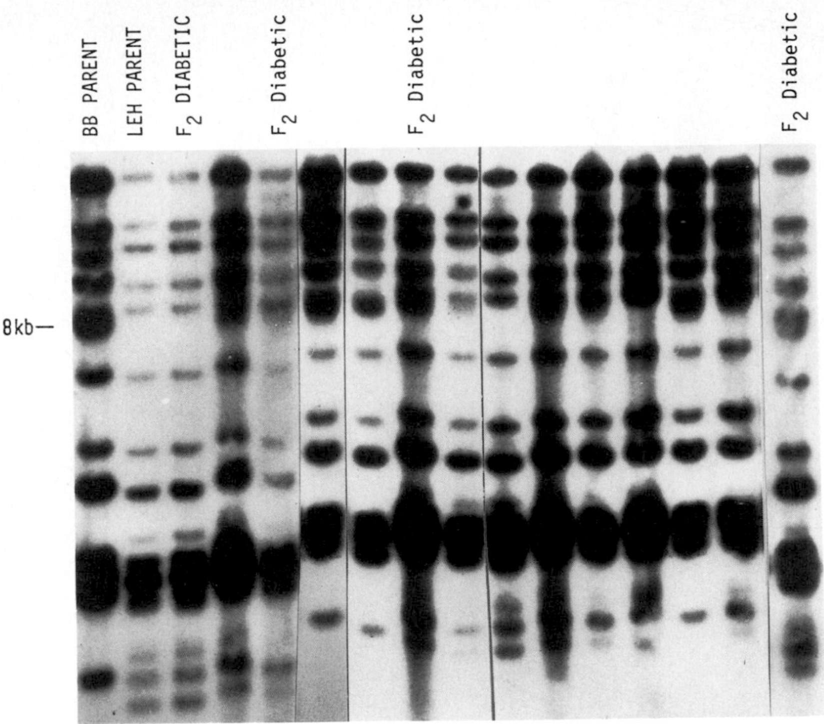

Msp I DIGESTION OF A CROSS

BETWEEN A DIABETIC BB AND A LONG EVANS HOODED

(probe = 4a22a)

Fig. 2. Msp I digestion of a cross between a diabetic BB and a Long Evans hooded rat (probe = 4a22a). Screening of a portion of the F_2 generation of a BB/H × Long Evans outcross for the presence of the 8-kb Msp RFLP. The *band* is seen as a doublet at 8 kilobases and is observed in the BB/H parent and three out of four diabetic F_2 animals while absent from the Long Evans parent

gel electrophoresis and Southern blotting. The presence or absence of the polymorphic band(s) was correlated with the inheritance of any of the disease traits (i.e., lymphopenia, diabetes, MHC haplotypes, age at onset, etc.). In this manner, the segregation of the RFLP with these traits was tested. The repetitive probe, 4a22a, which was described above, was used to hybridize to these blots. Among the many unlinked polymorphic loci that this probe detected was a band at 8kb. This band was present in five out of six of the diabetic F_2 animals, indicating a possible linkage to diabetes (Fig. 2). There did not seem to be linkage to the lymphopenia or MHC traits. If this observation represented true linkage, it detected a diabetes gene other than the MHC-linked or the lymphopenia gene. Further data has awaited the production of more diabetic F_2 animals through an additional cross between the BB and the Long Evans rats. Another repetitive

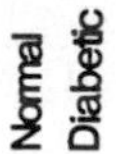

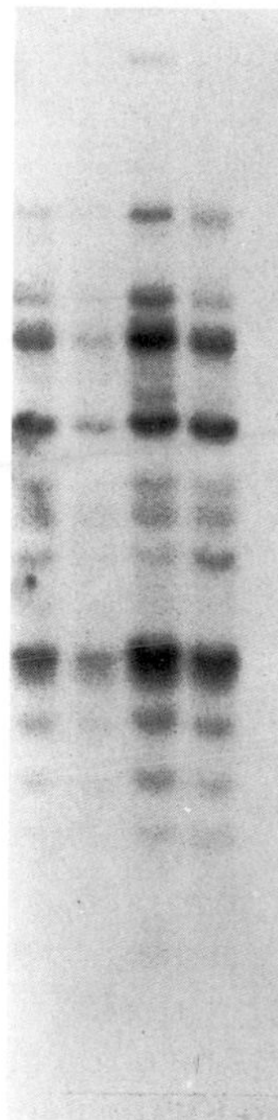

Fig. 3. The 2.3-kb RsaI fragment detected by a moderately repetitive rat DNA probe in the diabetes-resistant BB control line but absent in the diabetes-prone BB/H line

probe detected a 2.3-kb RsaI band which was missing in the diabetes-prone, BB/H, line, and present in the diabetes-resistant, BBC, line (Fig. 3). In the F_2 generation of a cross between these two animals, we observed that only 5/13 F_2 animals had the band. This was far less than the expected 10/13 for the inheritance of a dominant trait like an RFLP. If this was true linkage, it would indicate that the marker was located quite distal to the lymphopenia gene and would not be very useful except to identify which chromosome was involved. These promising, but preliminary, results demonstrate the usefulness of using random, repetitive DNA markers to detect linkage with the genes which lead to diabetes.

It is important to remember that these probes will probably not detect the actual diabetes genes. What they will detect are regions of a chromosome that are in proximity to the diabetes genes. The closeness of this linkage will be tested by assessing the frequency of recombination between the diabetes trait and the polymorphic locus that the probe detects.

The identification of the genes which lead to diabetes is merely the first step towards an understanding of the genetic mechanisms involved in the pathogenesis of the disease. After the identification of the chromosomal location of these genes, it may be possible to isolate the genes in question. The degree of difficulty involved in this will be determined by the relative proximity of the genes to the polymorphic markers. Short distances such as 1–2 cM may be spanned with relative ease by techniques such as chromosome walking. Longer distances would require more innovative approaches such as "jumping libraries" (Collins and Weissman 1984; Poustka and Lehrach 1986) or the identification of a genetic marker which is closer to the disease locus. The complexity of this task will be assessed when a successful linkage is determined.

4 Summary

Very little is known about the genes involved in the pathogenesis of IDDM. One component is known to be linked to the major histocompatibility complex, but the other components are unknown. We know from the major animals models of IDDM, both the NOD mouse and the BB rat, that the disease is under multigenic control. However, due to the size and complexity of the mammalian genome as well as to the lack of useful clues, the location and identity of the other genes remains a mystery. This is compounded by the fact that well-characterized genetic markers are not available for all regions of the mammalian genome, and it is likely that at least some of the genes of interest are located in these regions. The testing of pedigrees for the linkage of RFLP with the genetic factors involved in IDDM promises to be the most effective means of mapping, and ultimately identifying, these genes. However, the number of genes which are theoretically necessary to test for linkage makes even this approach impractical. Here, we have described here how the amount of work and time can be significantly reduced by utilizing repetitive DNA sequences as probes for the linkage of random RFLPs to diabetes. With each screening, one can simultaneously test multiple unlinked loci in the genome. Preliminary results which show promising linkage to two of the genetic components have been presented, thereby supporting the usefulness of this approach.

References

Bender K, Adams M, Baverstock PR, den Bieman M, Bissbort S, Brdicka R, Butcher GW, Cramer DV, von Deimling O, Festing MFW, Gunther E, Guttmann RD, Hedrich HJ, Kendall PB, Kluge R, Moutier R, Simon B, Womack JE, Yamada J, van Zutphen B (1984) Biochemical markers in inbred strains of the rat (*Rattus norvegicus*). Immunogenetics 19: 257–266

Bjørck L, Kryspin-Sørensen I, Dyrberg T, Lernmark A, Kastern W (1986) A deletion in a rat major histocompatibility complex class I gene is linked to the absence of beta$_2$-microglobulin-containing serum molecules. Proc Natl Acad Sci USA 83: 5630–5633

Botstein D, White RL, Skolnick M, Davis RW (1980) Construction of a genetic linkage map in man using restriction fragment length polymorphisms. Am J Hum Genet 32: 314–331

Britten R, Davidson EH (1969) Gene regulation for higher cells A theory. Science 165: 349–357

Britten R, Davidson EH (1971) Repetitive and non-repetitive DNA sequences and a speculation on the origins of evolutionary novelty. Q Rev Biol 46: 111–137

Colle E, Guttmann RD, Seemayer T (1981) Spontaneous diabetes mellitus syndrome in the rat. I. Association with the major histocompatibility complex. J Exp Med 154: 1237–1242

Colle E, Guttmann RD, Seemayer TA, Michel F (1983) Spontaneous diabetes mellitus syndrome in the rat. IV. Imunogenetic interactions of MHC and non-MHC components of the syndrome. Metabolism 32: 54–61

Colle E, Guttmann RD, Fuks A (1986) Insulin-Dependent diabetes mellitus is associated with genes that map to the right of the class I RT1. A locus of the major histocompatibility complex of the rat. Diabetes 35: 454–458

Collins FS, Weissman SM (1984) Directional cloning on DNA fragments at a large distance from an initial probe: circularization method. Proc Natl Acad Sci USA 81: 6812–6816

Davies KE (1981) The application of DNA recombinant technology to the analysis of the human genome and genetic disease. Hum Genet 58: 351–357

Deininger PL, Daniels GR (1986) The recent evolution of mammalian repetitive DNA elements. Trends Genet 2: 76–80

Gilliam TC, Tanzi RE, Haines JL, Bonner TI, Faryniarz AG, Hobbs AJ, MacDonald ME, Cheng SV, Folstein SE, Conneally PM, Wexler NS, Gusella JF (1987) Localization of the Huntington's disease gene to a small segment of chromosome 4 flanked by D4S10 and the telomere. Cell 50: 565–571

Guberski DL, Butler L, Kastern W, Like AA (1989) Genetic studies in inbred BB/Wor rats: analysis of progeny produced by crossing lymphopenic diabetes prone with non-lymphopenic rats. Diabetes (in press)

Gusella JF, Wexler NS, Conneally PM, Naylor SL, Anderson MA, Tanzi RE, Watkins PC, Ottina K, Wallace MR, Sakaguchi AY, Young AB, Shoulson I, Bonilla M, Martin JB (1983) A polymorphic DNA marker genetically linked to Huntington's disease. Nature 306: 234–239

Guttmann RD, Colle E, Michel F, Seemayer T (1983) Spontaneous diabetes mellitus syndrome in the rat. II. T lymphopenia and its association with clinical disease and pancreatic lymphocytic infiltration. J Immunol 130: 1732–1735

Hattori M, Buse JB, Jackson RA, Glimcher L, Dorf ME, Minami M, Makino S, Moriwaki K, Kuzuya H, Imura H, Strauss WM, Seidman JG, Eisenbarth G (1986) The NOD mouse: recessive diabetogenic gene in the major histocompatibility complex. Science 231: 733–735

Herold KC, Kastern W, Markholst H, Lernmark A (1989) Derivation of non-lymphopenic BB rats with an intercross breeding. Autoimmunity (in press)

Hill AVS, Jeffreys AJ (1985) Use of minisatellite DNA probes for determination of twin zygosity at birth. Lancet 2: 1394–1395

Holowachuk EW, Greer MK (1989) Unaltered class II histocompatibility antigens and pathogenesis of IDDM in BB rats. Diabetes 38: 267–271

Jackson RA, Buse JB, Rifai R, Pelletier D, Milford EL, Carpenter CB, Eisenbarth GS, Williams RM (1984) Two genes required for diabetes in BB rats. Evidence from cyclical intercrosses and backcrosses. J Exp Med 159: 1629–1636

Jeffreys AJ, Wilson V, Thein SL (1985a) Hypervariable 'minisatellite' regions in human DNA. Nature 314: 67–73

Jeffreys AJ, Brookfield JFY, Semeonoff R (1985b) Positive identification of one immigration test-case using human DNA fingerprints. Nature 317: 818–819

Jeffreys AJ, Wilson V, Thein SL, Weatherall DJ, Ponder BAJ (1986) DNA "Fingerprints" and segregation analysis of multiple markers in human pedigrees. Am J Hum Genet 39: 11–24

Jelinek W, Schmid CW (1982) Repetitive sequences in eukaryotic DNA and their expression. Annu Rev Biochem 51: 813–844

Knowlton RG, Cohen-Haguenauer O, Cong NV, Frezal J, Brown VA, Barker D, Braman JC, Schumm JW, Tsui LC, Buchwald M, Donis-Keller H (1985) A polymorphic DNA marker linked to cystic fibrosis is located in chromosome 7. Nature 318: 380–385

Kryspin-Sørensen I, Dyrberg T, Kastern W (1986) Genetic heterogeneity within the major histocompatibility complex of various BB rat sublines. Diabetologia 29: 307–312

Lang F, Kastern W (1989) The gene for the rat lymphocyte alloantigen is linked neither to diabetes nor lymphopenia and is apparently functional in the diabetic BB rat. Eur J Immunol (submitted)

Leiter E, Prochazka M (1988) Genetic loci controlling diabetes susceptibility in NOD mice. Diabetes Res. Clin Pract 5 [*suppl 1*]: S188

Like AA, Guberski DL, Butler L (1986) Diabetic BioBreeding/Worcestmr (BB/Wor) rats need not be lymphopenic. J Immunol 136: 3254–3258

Murray JM, Davies KE, Harper PS, Meredith L, Mueller CR, Williamson R (1982) Linkage relationship of a cloned DNA sequence on the short arm of the X chromosome to Duchenne muscular dystrophy. Nature 300: 69–71

O'Brien SJ (1987) *Genetic maps—1987*. Cold Spring Harbor Laboratory, New York

Ono SJ, Issa-Chergui B, Colle E, Guttmann RD, Seemayer TA, Fuks A (1988) Enhanced MHC class I heavy-chain gene expression in pancreatic islets. Diabetes 37: 1411–1418

Pearson WR, Wu JR, Bonner J (1978) Analysis of Rat Repetitive DNA sequences. Biochemistry 17: 51–59

Poussier P, Nakhooda AF, Falk J, Lee C, Marliss EB (1982) Lymphopenia and abnormal lymphocyte subsets in the "BB" rat: relationship to the diabetic syndrome. Endocrinology 110: 1825–1827

Poustka A, Lehrach H (1986) Jumping libraries and linking libraries: the next generation of molecular tools in mammalian genetics. Trends Genet 2: 174–179

Prochazka M, Leiter EH, Serreze DV, Coleman DL (1987) Three recessive loci required for insulin-dependent diabetes in nonobese diabetic mice. Science 237: 286–289

Rouleau GA, Wertelecki W, Haines JL, Hobbs WJ, Trofatter JA, Seizinger BR, Martuza RL, Superneau DW, Conneally PM, Gusella JF (1987) Genetic linkage of bilateral acoustic neurofibromatosis to a DNA marker on chromosome 22. Nature 329: 246–248

Schmid CW, Jelinek W (1982) The Alu family of dispersed repetitive sequences. Science 216: 1065–1070

Stock W, Gunther E (1979) Serologic analysis of two new alloantigenic systems of the rat major histocompatibility complex. Transplant Proc 11 (3): 1579–1581

White RL (1984) Human genetics. Lancet 2: 1257–1262

Wonigeit K, Hedrich HJ, Gunther E (1979) Serologic and histogenic analysis of apparently identical RTI haplotypes. Transplant Proc 11 (3): 1584–1586

Wyman AR, White R (1980) A highly polymorphic locus in human DNA. Proc Natl Acad Sci USA 77: 6574–6578

The Role of Class II Molecules in Development of Insulin-Dependent Diabetes Mellitus in Mice, Rats and Humans*

H. ACHA-ORBEA[1,2] and H. O. MCDEVITT[1]

1 Introduction

The major histocompatibility complex (MHC) represents a genetic risk factor for most known autoimmune diseases. More and more evidence implicates the class II region of the MHC in susceptibility in diseases such as insulin-dependent diabetes mellitus (IDDM), rheumatoid arthritis, and pemphigus vulgaris (for review see TODD et al. 1988). The gene products of this region are highly polymorphic and each individual expresses one or two alleles at each locus. Their function is the regulation of the immune response by binding fragments of proteins (peptides) with many different sequences and presenting them to the T cell receptor (TCR) which is expressed by T lymphocytes. Due to the polymorphism of class II molecules, each molecule binds a specific set of peptides (BUUS et al. 1987). These molecules are selective, but relatively nonspecific peptide receptors expressed on B lymphocytes, macrophages, and other cells collectively termed antigen presenting cells (APC'c) (UNANUE and ALLEN 1987). T cells expressing the surface marker CD4 represent the predominant type of T cells which interact with class II expressing cells. After formation of the trimolecular complex between TCR, MHC class II antigen, and peptide, T cell proliferation and differentiation is initiated.

It is not completely understood how an organism can distinguish between its own and foreign proteins. It has been clearly shown that the MHC cannot distinguish between self and foreign peptides. One of the critical sites of tolerance induction is located in the thymus. Strongly self-reactive T cells are eliminated (negative selection), while cells with less affinity towards self MHC (and peptide?) are positively selected (KAPPLER et al. 1987; KISIELOW et al. 1988). Therefore the palette of MHC alleles expressed in an organism shapes the repertoire of TCR molecules expressed in the periphery. The expressed repertoire of TCR as well as the MHC repertoire are important for establishing a state of tolerance. How and whether tolerance against peripheral self-antigens is achieved, or whether under

[1] Stanford University School of Medicine, Dept. of Medical Microbiology, Immunology and Medicine, Stanford CA 94305, USA

[2] Ludwig Institute for Cancer Research, CH-1066 Epalinges S. Lausanne, Switzerland

* The work was supported by NIH grant AIO07757 and H.A-O was supported by the Swiss National Science Foundation and the Juvenile Diabetes Foundation

Current Topics in Microbiology and Immunology, Vol. 156

normal conditions tolerance towards proteins expressed in immunologically privileged sites is required is not clear. In addition, suppression of immune responses in the periphery has been described, but the nature of the effector cell is unclear.

In an autoimmune disease an organism's own proteins are under attack by immune cells. Because the regulation of the immune response is highly complex, the possible reasons for this lack of self-tolerance are manifold.

One of at least three recessive susceptibility genes for IDDM in the nonobese diabetic (NOD) mouse maps to the MHC, most likely the class II molecule I-A (Acha-Orbea and McDevitt 1986, 1987; Hattori et al. 1986; Wicker et al. 1987; Prochazka et al. 1987). In the NOD mouse only I-A is expressed; the second class II antigen, I-E, cannot be expressed because no mRNA is detectable for the I-E α-chain (Hattori et al. 1986).

A very similar situation is found in humans where one of the susceptibility genes has been mapped to the class II region of the MHC. The class II region in humans can be divided into three subregions: DP, DQ and DR. Population analysis with a large sample showed that the DQ region (the human analogue of I-A) confers the highest risk of developing IDDM. In addition, expression of specific DQ antigens has a dominant protective effect on development of the disease (for review see Todd et al. 1988).

In the BioBreeding (BB) rat as well as a susceptibility gene maps to the MHC. Both class II antigens, RT1.B and RT1D are expressed and evidence for I-A/I-E hybrid proteins in autoimmune disease has been presented (Colle et al. 1981; Jackson et al. 1984; Naparstek et al. 1988; E. Heber Katz, personal communication). In the BB rat the region between RT1.A and RT1.C contains the susceptibility gene(s) (Colle et al. 1988).

Depletion of the CD4+ subset of T cell in NOD mice, and treatment with anticlass II antibodies in the rat and in mice prevents development of the spontaneous disease (Boitard et al. 1985, in press; Shizuru et al. 1988). In the BB rat addition of CD4+ or RT6+T cells prevents IDDM (Mordes et al. 1987; Greiner et al. 1987). Adoptive transfer studies in the NOD mouse implicated both the CD4 and CD8 subset of T cells in transfer of the disease; in rats it has been shown that the disease can be transferred with activated splenocytes (Miller et al. 1988; Bendelac et al. 1987; Koevary et al. 1983).

In light of these findings, we determined the cDNA sequences of the expressed class II antigens in all three systems in order to see whether specific class II sequences are found in diabetics. In the NOD mouse the I-A_α chain was identical to the previously published sequence of I-A^d but the I-A_β chain revealed a new allele in the first external domain of the molecule, whereas the rest of the molecule was identical to the previously published I-A^d sequence. This first external domain had 80%–90% amino acid homology to previously determined I-A_β sequences. The first external domains of the class II molecules are responsible for peptide binding and interaction with TCR. Most of the polymorphism is found in this region. The most striking observation in the NOD I-A_β sequence was a difference in a highly conserved region of the class II molecule: at positions 56 and

57 proline and aspartic acid were replaced by histidine and serine. All the other alleles had aspartic acid at position 57 and most alleles had proline at position 56 (ACHA-ORBEA and MCDEVITT 1986, 1987). Backcross studies indicated that the expression of one allele with aspartic acid at position 57 and/or proline at position 56 prevented development of the disease (HATTORI et al. 1986; WICKER et al. 1987; PROCHAZKA et al. 1987).

In humans, a very similar situation was encountered: The class II DQ_β genes which conferred risk of developing IDDM expressed serine, alanine or leucine at position 57, whereas the protective alleles expressed aspartic acid (TODD et al. 1987, 1988). Residue 57 of the $I\text{-}A_\beta$ and DQ_β chain seems to play the predominant role in mediating this effect. Other residues of the α- and β-chain, however, definitively contribute to susceptibility or resistance.

In the BB rat, no differences between the sequences of the susceptible and not susceptible rat strains were found. In all the alleles analyzed serine was found at position 57, which would allow development of the disease according to the results obtained in humans and in mice (TODD et al. 1988; CHAO et al. 1989). In the BB rat, therefore, other factors in the MHC also seem to influence susceptibility.

In this review we will give a short discussion of the role of class II antigens, present the class II sequencing results, and propose possible mechanisms by which the obtained results can be explained.

2 The Class II Region of the MHC

The MHC genes can be divided into three major regions: class I, II and III. The organization of the MHC and its nomenclature in mice, rats, and humans is shown in Fig. 1a. In humans this region is encoded on chromosome 6 and in mice on chromosome 17. The class II antigens of the MHC are heterodimeric glycoproteins consisting of an α and β chain, with molecular weights of 32 and 28 kDa respectively. Structurally, these proteins consists of two extracellular domains (α_1, α_2 and β_1, β_2), a transmembrane region, and a short cytoplasmatic tail (Fig. 1b). They are expressed on B lymphocytes, macrophages, and other cells collectively called antigen presenting cells (APCs). In human and rats they have been detected on activated T cells (MOELLER 1985).

The clsss II molecules are highly polymorphic and many different alleles have been described for each locus. Each individual expresses one or two alleles at each locus. The bulk of the amino acid differences between alleles resides in the first external domain of either chain (α_1, β_1). The alleles exhibit 1%–20% amino acid differences in this first external domain and the majority of amino acid differences are found clustered in three so-called allelic hypervariable regions. Comparison of a large number of sequences revealed that at each position in these

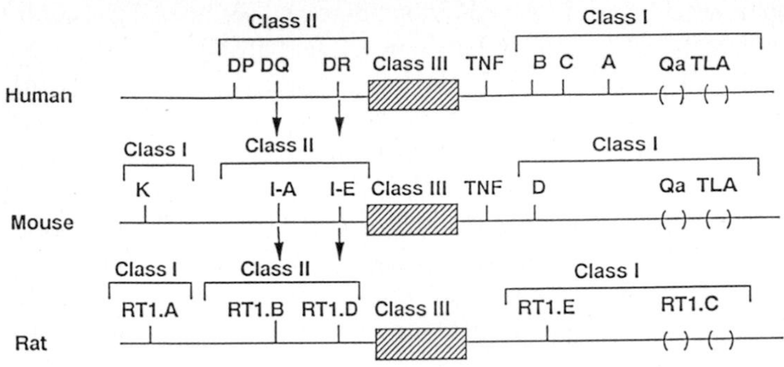

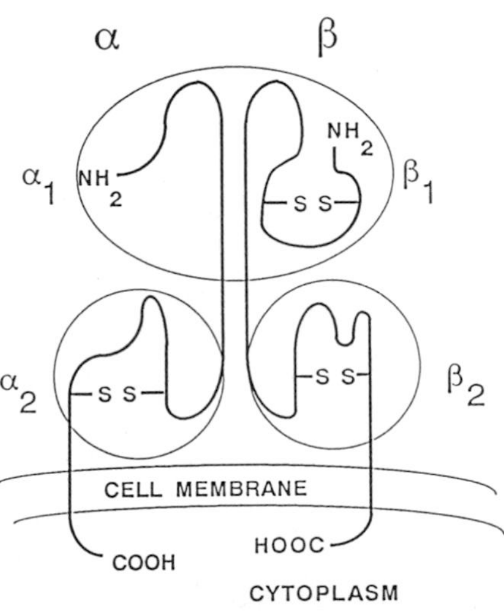

Fig. 1a. Genomic organization of the human, rat and mouse MHC comples. *Arrows* connect homologous class II loci. **b** Schematic structure of a class II molecule. (**b** from TODD et al. 1988)

hypervariable regions not more than four different amino acids are encountered (BELL et al., in press).

These molecules represent one of the sites where immune responses are regulated. The APCs process (degrade) foreign and self-proteins and some of the resultant peptide fragments are bound to MHC molecules and then transported to the cell surface. TCRs, expressed on the cell surface of T lymphocytes, recognize these complexes unless tolerance against class II and the antigen under study was induced. These cells are thus self-MHC restricted, i.e., recognize a foreign porten only when an immunogenic peptide is bound to self-MHC molecules (ZINKERNAGEL and DOHERTY 1979; BUUS et al. 1987). Class II molecules act as selective, but relatively nonspecific peptide receptors. They can

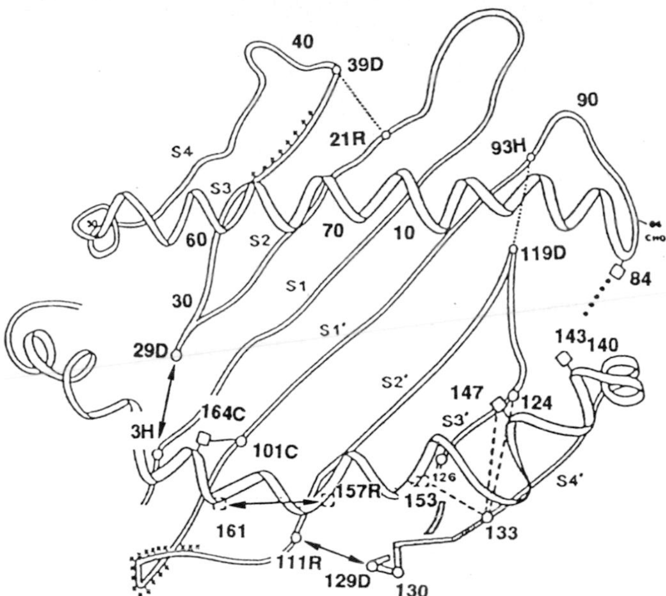

Fig. 2. Residues and intramolecular interactions which are shared by the HLA-A2 structure and the hypothetical class II structure. *Solid lines with arrows* indicate intramolecular salt bridges conserved in all class I and class II sequences. The *dotted line* between HLA-A2 residues *84* and *143* correspond to a Tyr-Thr salt bridge in class I molecules. This salt bridge could be formed in class II molecules with aspartic acid at position 57 of the β chain (143 in the class I structure). Residue *84* corresponds to arginine at position 79 of the class II α chain. In addition, the disulfide bridge between residues *101* and *164* of the HLA-A2 molecule and the hydrophobic cluster connected by *dashed lines* is conserved between class I and class II molecules. Shaded loops indicate similar residues in class I and class II molecules. Residue 86 is the common carbohydrate attachment site. Deletions and insertions in the class II sequence relative to HLA-A2 occur in loops S1-S2, S2-S3, S3-S4, H1'-H2' and at the N and C terminals of both α_1 and α_2 domains (from Brown et al. 1988)

bind a wide variety of peptide fragments including self-peptides, but every allele selects a specific set of peptides (Buus et al. 1987; Lorez and Allen 1988). The amino acid sequence differences between alleles are responsible for selecting which peptide fragments will be bound. Different peptide fragments can compete for binding on a particular class II molecule, arguing for a single peptide binding region in these molecules or for a conformational change after binding occurs (Guillet et al. 1987).

The crystal structure of a class I molecule, HLA-A2, has recently been determined (Bjorkman et al. 1987a, b). The extracellular domains fold together in such a way that a cleft is formed between the two external domains, with the majority of polymorphic amino acids pointing towards its center. It appears that this cleft represents the peptide binding groove. Class I and II antigens are likely to be structurally similar, and a model structure for class II molecules has been proposed based on the crystal structure of HLA-A2 (see Fig. 2), (Brown et al. 1988).

3 Induction of Self-Tolerance

MHC class II antigens cannot distinguish between foreign and self-peptides (Lorenz and Allen 1988). These molecules may represent one level of prevention of self-recognition by determinant selection, but other mechanisms must be present as well. The thymus represents the site where self-tolerance is induced. Good evidence for positive selection (selection of TCR molecules which can interact with self-MHC molecules) and negative selection (elimination of T cell which interact too strongly with self-MHC or self-MHC and self-peptide) has been presented (Kappler et al. 1987; Kisielow et al. 1988). Therefore the class II antigens shape the expressed repertoire of TCR. In addition, regulation of the response towards self-molecules in the periphery has been reported. The mechanism of tolerance induction towards proteins expressed only in the periphery is still not understood.

4 IDDM in Mice, Rats, and Humans

The disease in the two animal models for IDDM, the NOD mouse and the BB rat and in humans exhibits similarities as well as differences. Some of the characteristics of the disease are shown in Table 1.

The disease is clearly autoimmune mediated in all three species and one of the susceptibility genes has been mapped to the MHC (Colle et al. 1981; Hattori et al. 1986; Todd et al. 1988). In humans and mice the DQ or I-A region of the MHC seems to represent a disease susceptibility locus (Acha-Orbea et al. 1986, 1987; Todd et al. 1987, 1988). Population studies revealed in humans that dominant protection is conferred by specific DQ alleles, such as DQw3.1,

Table 1. Insulin-dependent diabetes in humans, NOD mice and BB rats

	NOD mouse	Humans	BB rat
Glycosuria and ketosis	+	+	+
Insulin dependence	+	+	+
Age of onset	Early adolescence	Puberty	Early adolescence
Female:male ratio	1.5–10	1	1
Role of MHC	+	+	+
Number of genes involved	$\geqslant 3$	$\geqslant 1$	$\geqslant 2$
Lymphopenia	–	–	+
Autoantibodies to islet cells	+	+	+
Predominant role of T cells	+	+?	+
Requirement for exogenous agents	–	?	–
Role of exogenous agents	+	+	+
Insulitits	+	+	+

DQw1.12, DQw1.2, DQw1.18, DQw1.9, and DQwBlank, whereas in subject with IDDM, DQw3.2, DQw2, DQw1.1, DQw1.19 and DQw1. AZH are found in most cases on both alleles (for review see TODD et al 1988). In humans, several different DQ alleles are found in diseased individuals, so that susceptibility is therefore not recessive in a classical way. In addition, the vast majority of individuals expressing two susceptibility alleles never develop the disease. In NOD mice dominant protection H-2^b, H-2^k, and H^{NON} has been found (HATTORI et al. 1986; PROCHAZKA et al. 1987; WICKER et al. 1987).

A diabetes prone and a diabetes resistant subline of the BB rat have been derived (for review see ROSSINI et al. 1985). After backcrossing Wistar Furth, Buffalo, or Lewis rats with diabetes prone BB rats, the majority of animals with IDDM expressed two copies of the class II genes of the BB rat (COLLE et al. 1981; JACKSON et al. 1984). Nevertheless diabetic heterozygotes were found more frequently than in humans and in the NOD mouse (COLLE et al. 1983). In both humans (5%–10%) and NOD mice (0%–5%) a minority of diseased individuals express one protective allele. It was not excluded however, whether the disease in heterozygous NOD animals resulted from a recombination element. Diabetes in homozygotes for protective alleles is very rare and has never been found in mice (WICKER and MILLER 1988; TODD et al. 1988).

These results point to a complex form of inheritance on the disease, but highlight the similarities between mouse and man. Besides the MHC, which carries a susceptibility gene in all three systems, other genes are required for induction of the disease. In mice, using different strain combinations at least one dominant and two other recessive susceptibility genes have been detected. Besides the one which was localized in the MHC, another could be mapped close to the Thy-1 locus on chromosome 9 (PROCHAZKA et al. 1987). In humans there is evidence that at least one and perhaps several genes other than the gene(s) mapping to the MHC are involved in mediating susceptibility. The concordance rate for monozygotic twins is about 30%–50%, which indicates that environmental factors contribute significantly to disease development. Sib pair analysis of siblings expressing the same MHC genes revealed a concordance rate of about 10%–15% (ROTTER and LANDAU 1984). The difference can be explained most easily by postulating other unmapped susceptibility genes. In rats a gene which is responsible for mediating lymphopenia, the absence of a subset of T cells expressing the RT6 marker, represents a second susceptibility gene (COLLE et al. 1983; JACKSON et al. 1984; GREINER et al. 1986), however, a very small percentage of animals with IDDM can be detected without lymphopenia (LIKE et al. 1986).

In both rats and mice, the disease can be transfered into healthy animals with T lymphocytes obtained from sick animals. In mice it was demonstrated that both CD4 + and CD8 + T cells need to be transfered from a sick animal to a healthy animal to transfer the disease, and in rats it was shown that activated splenocytes obtained from rats with IDDM transfered the disease (KOEVARY et al. 1983; BENDELAC et al. 1987; MILLER et al. 1988). Mixing one subset of T cells from young NOD mice with the other from diseased animals did not result in IDDM. Allogeneic bone marrow chimeras, thymectomy, and, in the rat, the addition of RT6 + T cells prevented the development of the disease. In rats it is not clear what population of T cells is involved in pathogenesis, but Natural Killer (NK) cells have been implicated (WODA and BIRON 1986). The RT6 + T cells seems to have a regulatory function since depletion of the RT6 + cells from diabetes resistant BB rats results in susceptibility (GREINER et al. 1987).

The disease can be prevented by depletion of CD4 + T cells in mice and in both rats and mice by administration of anticlass II monoclonal antibodies (BOITARD et al. 1985, 1988; SHIZURU et al. 1988). In addition, in all three species treatment with cyclosporine A prevents or, if given very early after diagnosis, reverts disease.

Lymphokines clearly play a role in pathogenesis in the NOD mouse. The gene encoding tumor necrosis factor (TNF) α is encoded within the MHC (MUELLER et al. 1987; CARROLL et al. 1987). NOD mice produce lower than average levels of TNF-α or interleukin-1 (IL-1) upon mitogen stimulation of immune cells. Although it has been reported that IL-1 is toxic for islet cells in vitro and that TNF-α has a synergistic effect, administration of either of these two lymphokines in vivo prevents insulitis and disease (BENDTZEN et al. 1986; PUJOL-BORRELL et al. 1987; CAMPBELL et al. 1988; JACOB et al., in press).

5 Sequence Analysis of Class II Genes

In order to determine whether unique class II sequences are found exclusively in individuals with IDDM or whether specific sequences associated with a risk of developing IDDM are found in sick as well as in normal individuals, cDNA sequences of all expressed class II alleles in humans, NOD mice, and the BB rat were determined. The results are displayed in Fig. 3. In the NOD mouse, a unique disease sequence was found which was not present or very rare in the normal mouse population. The only unique feature of this sequence was the difference to the previously determined cDNA sequences of the I-A_β chain at amino acid positions 56 and 57. In this stretch of highly conserved amino acid sequence, proline and aspartic acid were replaced by histidine and serine (see Fig. 3; ACHA-ORBEA and MCDEVITT 1986, 1987). The sequence of I-A_β of the nonobese nondiabetic (NON) mouse strain, a strain separated from NOD after the sixth inbreeding generation, shared the allelic hypervariable region after residue 57, but expressed aspartic acid at position 57 (TODD et al. 1988). In humans a very similar situation was found in the DQ_β chain. All the alleles found frequently in diabetics had alanine, valine, or serine at position 57, whereas the protective sequences had the charged residue aspartic acid. These sequences, however, are found in a large proportion of healthy individuals (TODD et al. 1987, 1988; MOREL et al. 1988). In the BB rat no differences between the susceptible and the nonsusceptible BB rat strains were detected in the β chains. Both the I-A and I-E homologue RT1.B and RT1.D were identical. In either strain, residue 57 of the

	Association with IDDM	2	3	9	12	13	14	26	28	30	37	38	40	45	46	47	52	53	55	56	57	61	63	65	66	67	70	71	74	75	77	78	84	85	86	87	88	89	90
A_β^{NOD}	+	D	S	H	K	G	E	L	T	Y	Y	L	F	G	E	Y	E	L	R	H	S	Y	K	*	Y	*	R	T	E	L	T	A	E	E	T	E	V	P	T
A_β^{b}	-	-	-	Y	M	-	-	Y	-	-	-	V	Y	-	-	H	-	-	-	P	D	W	S	P	E	I	-	-	-	-	-	V	-	G	P	-	T	H	-
A_β^{k}	-	N	-	-	Q	P	F	-	I	-	-	V	-	-	-	-	-	-	-	P	D	W	-	*	-	*	-	-	-	-	-	V	-	K	-	-	T	-	-
A_β^{NON}	-							S	-	N	-	-	Y	-	-	-	-	-	-	S	D	F	-	*	-	*	Q	-	A	-	-	V							
DQ_βw1.2 (DR2)	-	D	-	F	-	-	M	-	-	-	-	A	-	-	V	-	P	Q	-	P	D	W	S	K	E	V	G	-	-	-	-	V	-	V	A	F	R	G	I
DQ_βw1.12 (DR2)	0-	D	P	L	-	A	M	Y	-	-	D	V	-	-	V	-	P	Q	-	P	D	W	S	K	D	I	-	-	-	-	-	V	-	V	A	F	R	G	I
DQ_βw3.1 (DR4,5,w8)	0-	D	-	Y	-	A	M	Y	-	-	-	A	-	E	V	-	P	-	P	P	D	W	S	K	E	V	-	-	-	-	-	V	Q	L	E	L	R	T	-
DQ_βwBlank (DR4)	0	D	-	F	-	-	M	G	-	-	-	A	-	-	V	-	P	-	-	L	D	W	S	K	D	I	E	D	S	V	-	V	Q	L	E	L	R	T	-
DQ_βw1.1 (DR1)	+	D	-	Y	-	-	L	G	-	H	-	V	-	-	V	-	P	Q	-	P	V	W	S	K	E	V	G	A	S	V	R	V	-	V	A	Y	R	G	I
DQ_βw1.AZH (DR2)	+	D	-	Y	-	-	L	G	-	H	-	V	-	-	V	-	P	Q	-	P	S	W	S	K	E	V	G	A	S	V	R	V	-	V	A	Y	R	G	I
DQ_β1.19 (DRw6)	+	D	-	Y	-	-	M	-	-	H	-	A	-	-	V	-	P	Q	-	P	V	W	S	K	E	V	-	-	-	-	-	V	-	V	G	Y	R	G	I
DQ_βw2 (DR3,7)	+	D	-	Y	-	-	M	-	S	S	I	V	-	-	-	F	L	-	L	P	A	W	S	K	D	I	-	K	A	V	R	V	Q	L	E	L	R	T	-
DQ_βw3.2 (DR4)	+	D	-	Y	-	-	M	-	-	-	-	A	-	-	V	-	P	-	L	P	A	W	S	K	E	V	-	-	-	-	-	V	Q	L	E	L	R	T	-
RT1.B_β^{u}	+	R	L	V	-	P	Y	N	I	-	-	-	Y	-	-	-	-	-	G	P	-	F	-	*	-	*	-	-	-	-	-	V	-	K	-	-	-	-	-
RT1.D_β^{u}	+	-	P	G	-	F	-	-	A	L	-	A	-	-	-	-	-	-	G	P	-	R	-	K	E	F	-	R	A	V	-	Y	-	I	F	D	R	F	L

Fig. 3. Comparison of polymorphic class II amino acid sequences involved in susceptibility or protection from IDDM from humans, mice, and rats (Acha-Orbea and McDevitt 1987; Todd et al. 1987, 1988; Bell et al. 1989; Chao et al. 1989). The *asterisk* denotes a deletion of one amino acid; *dashes* indicate an identical amino acid residue as in the NOD sequence

RT1.B and RT1.D β chain was a serine, which would, according to the human and mouse situation, allow development of IDDM. Also, other rat class II alleles expressed serine at position 57 (CHAO et al. 1989). If this hypothesis is correct, other closely linked genes or different amino acid residues in the BB rat RT1.B_β or RT1.D_β chain are responsible for the development of the disease (BOITARD et al. 1985).

It seems obvious that this one amino acid is not the only difference responsible between the different alleles important for the development of the disease. However, residue 57 represents the only residue which clearly distinguishes susceptibility and protection. Other amino acids in the DQ_β chain and the sequences found in the α chain also contribute to the overall role of the class II molecule. In agreement with this, several exceptions to the rule are found. The majority of caucasian DR7 expressing individuals express DQw2, the DQ_β chain coexpressed with DR3. Although DR3 individuals are frequently found in the diabetes population, DR7 is not increased in IDDM (TODD et al. 1988). Other residues or a contribution of the unique DR7 linked DQ_α chain may be responsible. TODD et al. recently showed that different DQ_α chains associated with DQw2 in the DR7 haplotype lead to increased susceptibility (TODD et al. 1989). Clearly residue 57 represents only one of probably multiple residues important for development of the disease.

6 Possible Mechanisms

In the NOD mouse, the I-A molecules is the only class II molecule expressed (HATTORI et al. 1986). The sequencing results in both humans and the NOD mouse, together with the previous mapping of the susceptibility gene closest to the DQ subregion, makes this gene the best candidate for one of the susceptibility genes (ACHA-ORBEA and MCDEVITT 1986, 1987; TODD et al. 1987, 1988). In addition, the function of these molecules lies in the regulation of the immune response, and therefore it is easy to envision how these molecules are important in an autoimmune response.

How can one amino acid change have such a profound effect on susceptibility to IDDM? A model for the structure of class II molecules based on the known crystal structure of the HLA-A2 class I molecule suggests that residue 57 of the I-A_β or DQ_β chain is located at the end of the peptide binding groove (see Fig. 2; BROWN et al. 1988). In addition, this residue is pointing into the assumed peptide binding site. Having aspartic acid at this position could allow the formation of a salt bridge with arginine which is located at the end of the α-helix of the DQ_α or I-A_α chain. Therefore, an amino acid substitution in position 57 in the β chain can have a profound effect on the shape of the peptide binding groove and thereby influence the peptide binding pattern and/or TCR recognition of the MHC molecule. This could explain such a profound effect. Nevertheless, other allelic differences are likely to play an important role in peptide binding as well.

6.1 Mechanisms Which May Explain Dominant Protection and Recessive Susceptibility Class II Linked Mediated by a Gene

6.1.1 Selection in the Thymus

The expressed MHC antigens shape the repertoire of expressed TCR molecules by two mechanisms, called positive and negative selection in the thymus (KAPPLER et al. 1987; KISIELOW et al. 1988). The protective class II antigens which express aspartic acid at position 57, but not alleles with an uncharged residue, may negatively select a population of TCR molecules which are required for the destruction of the islet cells of the pancreas. Alternatively, by positive selection of a regulatory cell which is involved in protection from destruction of the islet cells, protection would also be obtained.

In a similar manner other MHC genes can have a modulatory effect on development of disease. In addition, these selection mechanisms may explain complexities in the genetic analysis of susceptibility. The negative selection hypothesis may help to understand the observations made by Kishimoto and coworkers (NISHIMOTO et al. 1987). By breeding a transgenic C57BL/6 mouse expressing an I-E_α transgene with NOD mice, they found after several backcrosses that these mice are not prone to insulitis and disease. They argued that I-E represents the protective gene mapping to the MHC and that it functions by induction of suppressor T cells. The results from backcross studies of NOD mice with normal C57/BL6 mice, which both lack a functional I-E_α gene and therefore cannot express I-E antigens, still indicated a recessive gene mapping to the MHC (WICKER et al. 1987). Therefore, I-E represents a second independent factor for protection from IDDM in NOD mice.

One of the key findings in demonstrating negative selection was that mouse strains which express I-E molecules clonally delete T cells expressing TCR molecules with the variable elements $V_\beta 11$, $V_\beta 17$, and possibly others (KAPPLER et al. 1987; E. PALMER, personal communication). Therefore, one of the reasons why these I-E_α transgenic mice do not develop disease is that they may eliminate specific populations of T cells in the thymus which by coincidence are the autoimmune T cells involved in development of IDDM. A very limited heterogeneity of TCR molecules involved in another autoimmune disease, experimental allergic encephalomyelitis (EAE), has recently been described (ACHA-ORBEA et al. 1988).

In preliminary experiments in the NOD mouse, adoptive transfer of T cells depleted of cells expressing the TCR V_β regions $V_\beta 6$, $V_\beta 8$, or $V_\beta 11$ failed to prevent the transfer of the disease ($V_\beta 17$ is not expressed in NOD mice; H. ACHA-ORBEA, unpublished observations). These results, however, do not disprove the mechanism because (1) a different V region could be used predominantly in IDDM and (2) the heterogeneity of TCR used in an autoimmune response need not to be similarly heterogeneous in early stages and in late stages of the disease.

6.1.2 Cross Tolerance

A frequent finding with antigen specific, MHC-restricted T cell clones is crossreactivity with allo-MHC molecules or allorestriction with the same or different antigens. Individuals are generally tolerant to their own MHC molecules. Therefore tolerance to protective class II molecules, but not to the alleles found in IDDM could by coincidence inactivate or deplete a population of autoimmune T cells required for pathogenesis. Induction of tolerance to (NODxBALB/c)F1 MHC antigens decreased the incidence of diabetes in NOD mice (CARNAUD et al. 1988).

6.1.3 Suppression

Different DQ or I-A antigens may have a different ability to suppress an immune response. DQ molecules have been implicated in suppression by several studies (HIRAYAMA et al. 1987; FESTENSTEIN and OLLIER 1987). In the NOD mouse evidence for lack of suppression in IDDM has been described (SERREZE and LEITER 1988). Therefore, DQ or I-A molecules with aspartic acid at position 57 should be more effective in inducing suppression than molecules without a negative charge at this position. Treatment of NOD mice with an anticlass II monoclonal antibody permitted the development of T cells capable of suppressing adoptive transfer of IDDM with diabetic NOD spleen cells (BOITARD et al. 1988).

6.1.4 Levels of Expression

At present it is not clear how the expression levels of different class II molecules in different organs are regulated. Different expression levels at critical sites (aberrant expression) or at sites critical for tolerance induction of aspartic acid positive and negative class II molecules could explain the results mentioned above. Evidence of tissue specific increased expression of class II molecules at the site of the autoimmune reaction in strains of rats and mice susceptible to experimental allergic encephalomyelitis has been presented (MASSA et al. 1987).

6.1.5 Molecular Mimicry

An exogenous antigen can activate T cells in the periphery which then may crossreact to islet cell antigens. In EAE in rats, it has been shown that activated cells of any specificity can enter the brain, a well-known privileged site from the immune system. If these T cells encounter a stimulatory antigen an autoimmune response then ensues (WEKERLE et al., personal communication). A similar situation might be found in IDDM, where autoimmune T cells may be activated by encountering a crossreactive exogenous antigen in the periphery.

7 The BB Rat

In all rat class II β chain sequences analyzed so far, serine was found at position 57 (CHAO et al. 1989). Expression of serine would allow the establishment of IDDM based on the above mentioned hypothesis. In rats, at least one susceptibility allele in the class II region is required. Although the majority of rats with IDDM are homozygous for the BB RT1^{u} class II genes, a higher proportion of diabetic heterozygous animals at the class II region is found than in humans and NOD mice. Therefore, if the hypothesis is correct, another gene in close linkage to the rat class II antigens might be responsible for susceptibility. The susceptibility gene(s) has been mapped between RT1.A and RT1.C. In both humans and mice, TNF-α is encoded in this region. Heterozygous animals would then express intermediate levels of this lymphokine and therefore exhibit an intermediate susceptibility. At present nothing is known about TNF-α levels in diabetes prone rats and possibly other immunoregulatory genes are encoded in this region. Other unknown factors are the relative expression levels of RT1.B and RT1.D in diabetes prone and resistant rats. Again, F1 animals would express intermediate levels and may contribute to susceptibility according to one of these mechanisms.

8 Future Prospects

Although there is good evidence that the class II antigens, represent susceptibility genes for IDDM and that residue 57 in the β chain is important for disease development, this needs to be confirmed by analysis of large numbers of diabetics and controls. In one such study the relative risk of developing IDDM increased from 8 to 107.5 when groups not expressing aspartic acid at position 57 of the DQ_{β} chain were analyzed (MOREL et al. 1988). In addition, it should be shown in direct experiments that this residue is crucial for disease development. The NOD mouse allows the design of such experiments. We are in the process of producing transgenic mice with I-A antigens. Introduction of an I-A_{β} molecule other than I-A_{β}^{NOD} should prevent IDDM; I-A_{β}^{NOD} should have no effect; and I-A_{β}^{NOD} with an amino acid substitution at position 57 (from serine to aspartic acid) should prevent the disease. Preliminary experiments failed because introduction of the I-A_{β} chain without the α chain resulted in transgenic mice with limited life expectancy (H. ACHA-ORBEA et al., unpublished observations).

IDDM clearly is a very complex disease, and many different pathogenic processes contribute to disease development. The search for a deeper understanding of the disease process, for tools enabling risk groups to be predicted with greater accuracy, and finally the search for a way to prevent the disease are all under way. Class II antigens play a central role in the pathogenesis. Several approaches to trying to influence the disease process are possible, and the NOD mouse and the BB rat serve as genetically well-defined model systems. The search has begun for peptides which do not elicit an autoimmune response but can prevent the induction of autoimmune responses by blocking class II active sites or inducing suppression of an immune response. Alternatively, antibodies directed at I-A or DQ molecules not expressing aspartic acid could block an autoimmune response.

To develop IDDM in mice, rats, and humans, several genetic requirements have to be fulfilled. Knowledge of the genetic factors in and outside the MHC would permit definition of risk groups with much greater accuracy.

Cyclosporine A has a preventive effect on development of IDDM in humans, rats, and mice (Bougeneres et al. 1988). Unfortunately, this drug has serious side effects in patients after long-term treatment. Other reagents which influence the immune system with less toxic side effects for the patient must be found.

Lymphokines are appearing to be more and more important in many autoimmune diseases. Administration of interferon-γ often exacerbates autoimmune diseases, whereas TNF-α has a beneficial effect in most diseases studied (Segiescu et al. 1979; Engelman et al. 1981; Parsitol et al. 1986; Jacob and McDevitt 1988; Jacob et al., in press). In NOD mice, low levels of IL-1, IL-2, and TNF-α have been found and treatment with IL-1, IL-2 or TNF-α prevented the onset of the disease in NOD mice (Jacob et al., in press; E.H. Leiter, personal communication). It remains to be determined what these lymphokines do in vivo, and whether short-term exposure at a crucial point in time allows prevention or reversal of the disease. Finally, depletion of activated T cells with anti-IL-2 receptor antibodies, elimination of the CD4-population of T cells, and treatment with anticlass II antibodies prevent the disease in NOD mice (Boitard et al. 1985, 1988; Shizuru et al. 1988; Kelley et al. 1988). Although these forms of immune intervention are not very specific for autoimmune T cells, these observations are highly encouraging.

Another important goal is the characterization of the islet cell antigens which elicit the initial autoimmune response. Knowledge of the heterogeneity of antigens involved in this process could help define specific and direct preventive tools. This would open the door to other means of intervention, such as tolerance induction or analysis of the heterogeneity of TCR molecules involved in the autoimmune process. While IDDM is a complex disease process, it is subject to attack at several critical points. The prospects for eventual prevention of this disease are therefore quite promising.

Acknowledgments. We thank Ed Palmer and Ellen Heber-Katz for providing us with information prior to publication.

References

Acha-Orbea H, McDevitt HO (1986) The cDNA-sequence of the I-A major histocompatibility antigens of the non-obese diabetic mouse. In: Jaworsky MA, Molnar GD, Rajotte RV, Singh B (eds) Excerpta Medica international congress series: immunology of diabetes. Excerpta Medica, Amsterdam, pp 73–78

Acha-Orbea H, McDevitt HO (1987) The first external domain of the non-obese diabetic mouse class II A_β chain is unique. Proc Natl Acad Sci USA 84: 2435–2439

Acha-Orbea H, Mitchell DJ, Timmermann L, Wraith DC, Tausch GS, Waldor MK, Zamvil SS, McDevit HO, Steinman L (1988) Limited heterogeneity of T cell receptors from lymphocytes mediating autoimmune encephalomyelitis allows specific immune intervention. Cell 54: 263–273

Bell JI, Todd JA, McDevitt HO (1989) The molecular basis of HLA disease associations. In: Harris H, Hirschhanl K (eds) Advances of human genetics. Vol. 18 Plenum Press New York, pp 1–35

Bendelac A, Carnaud C, Boitard C, Bach JF (1987) Syngeneic transfer of autoimmune diabetes from diabetic NOD mice to healthy neonates. Requirements for both L3T4 + and Lyt-2 + T cells. J Exp Med 166: 823–832

Bendtzen K, Mandrup-Poulsen T, Nerup J, Nielsen JH, Dinarello CA, Svenson M (1986) Cytotoxicity of human p17 interleukin-1 for pancreatic islets of langerhans. Science 232: 1545–1547

Bjorkman PJ, Saper MA, Samraoui B, Bennett WS, Strominger JL, Wiley DC (1987a) The foreign antigen binding site and T cell recognition regions of class I histocompatibility antigens. Nature 329: 512–518

Bjorkman PJ, Saper MA, Samraoui B, Bennett WS, Strominger JL, Wiley DC (1987b) Structure of the human class I histocompatibility antigen, HLA-A2. Nature 329: 506–512

Boitard C, Michie S, Serrurier P, Butcher GW, Larkins AP, McDevitt HO (1985) In vivo prevention of thyroid and pancreatic autoimmunity in the BB rat by antibody to class II major histocompatibility complex gene products. Proc Natl Acad Sci USA 82: 6627–6631

Boitard C, Bendelac A, Richard MF, Carnaud C, Bach JF (1988) Prevention of diabetes in non obese diabetic mice by abti-I-A monoclonal antibodies; transfer of protection by splenic T cells. Proc Natl Acad Sci USA 85: 9719–9723

Bougeneres PF, Carel JC, Castaneo L, Boitard C, Gardin JP, Laandais P, Hors J, Mihatsch MJ, Paillard M, Chaussain JL, Bach JF (1988) Factors associated with early remission of type I diabetes in children treated with cyclosporine. N Engl J Med 318: 663–670

Brown JH, Jardetzky T, Saper MA, Samraoui B, Bjorkman PJ, Wiley DC (1988) A hypothetical model of the foreign antigen binding site of class II histocompatibility molecules. Nature 332: 845–850

Buus S, Sette A, Grey HM (1987) The interaction between protein derived immunogenic peptides and la. Immunol Rev 98: 115–141

Campbell IL, Iscaro A, Harrison LC (1988) Ifn-γ and tumor necrosis factor-α. Cytotoxicity to murine islets of langerhans. J Immunol 141: 2325–2329

Carnaud C, Bendelac A, Boitard C, Bach JF (1988) Failure to induce neonatal tolerance in the autoimmune nonobese diabetic (NOD) mouse strain. Diabetes 37: 1A

Carroll MC, Katzman P, Alicot EM, Koller BH, Geraghty DE, Orr HT, Strominger SL, Spies T (1987) Linkage map of the human major histocompatibility complex including the tumor necrosis factor genes. Proc Natl Acad Sci USA 84: 8535–8539

Chao NJ, Timmerman L, McDevitt HO, Jacob CO (1989) Molecular characterization of MHC class II antigens (β_1 domain) in the BB diabetes prone and resistant rat. Immunogenetics 29: 231–234

Colle E, Gurrmann RD, Seemayer T (1981) Spontaneous diabetes mellitus syndrome in the rat I. Association with the major histocompatibility complex. J Exp Med 154: 1237–1242

Colle E, Guttmann RD, Seemayer TA, Michel F (1983) Spontaneous diabetes mellitus syndrome in the rat IV. Immunogenetic interactions of MHC and non-MHC components in the syndrome. Metabolism 32: 54–61

Colle E, Ono SJ, Fuks A, Guttmann RD, Seemayer TA (1988) Association of susceptibility to spontaneous diabetes in rat with genes of major histocompatibility complex. Diabetes 37: 1438–1443

Engelman EG, Sonnenfeld G, Dauphinee M, Greenspan JS, Talal J, McDevitt HO (1981) Treatment of NZB/NZW F1 mice with mycobacterium bovis strain BCG or type II interferon preparations accelerates autoimmune disease. Arthritis Rheum 24: 1396

Festenstein H, Ollier B (1987) Cellulasr typing and functional heterogeneity of MHC-encoded products. Br Med Bull 43: 122–155

Greiner DL, Handler ES, Nakano K, Mordes JP, Rossini AA (1986) Absence of the RT-6 T-cell subset in diabetes prone BB/W rats. J Immunol 136: 148–151

Greiner DL, Mordes JP, Handler ES, Angelillo M, Nakamura N, Rossini AA (1987) Depletion of RT6.1 + T lymphocytes induces diabetes in resistant biobreeding/Worcester (BB/W) rats. J Exp Med 166: 461–475

Guillet JG, Lai MZ, Briner TJ, Buus S, Sette A, Grey HM, Smith JA, Gefter ML (1987) Immunological self, non-self discrimination. Science 235: 865–870
Hattori M, Buse JB, Jackson RA, Glimcher L, Dorf ME, Minami M, Makino S, Moriwaki K, Kuzuya H, Imura H, Strauss WM, Seidman JG, Eisenbarth GS (1986) The NOD mouse: recessive diabetogenic gene in the major histocompatibility complex. Science 231: 733–735
Hirayama K, Matsushita S, Kihashi I, Iuchi M, Ohta N, Sasazuki T (1987) HLA-DQ is epistatic to HLA-DR in controlling the immune response to schistosomal antigen in humans. Nature 327: 426–430
Jackson RA, Buse JB, Rifai R, Pelletier D, Milford EL, Carpenter CB, Eisenbarth GS, Williams M (1984) Two genes required for fiabetes in BB rats. Evidence from cyclical intercrosses and backcrosses. J Exp Med 159: 1629–1636
Jacob CO, McDevitt HO (1988) Tumor necrosis factor-α in murine autoimmune "lupus" nephritis. Nature 331: 356–358
Jacob CO, Aiso S, Michie SA, McDevitt HO, Acha-Orbea H (1990) Tumor necrosis factor in autoimmunity: protective effect on non-obese diabetic mice. Proc Natl Acad Sci US, in press
Kappler JW, Roehm N, Marrack P (1987) T cell tolerance by clonal elimination in the thymus. Cell 49: 273–280
Kelley VE, Gaulton GN, Hattori M, Ikegami H, Eisenbarth G, Strom TB (1988) Anti-interleukin 2 receptor antibody suppresses murine diabetic insulitis and lupus nephritis. J Immunol 140: 59–61
Kisielow P, Teh HS, Bluethmann H, vonBoehmer H (1988) Positive selection of antigen apecific T cells by restricting MHC molecules. Nature 335: 730–733
Koevary S, Rossini AA, Stoller W, Chick WL, Williams RM (1983) Passive transfer of diabetes in the BB/W rat. Science 220: 727–728
Like AA, Guberski DL, Butler L (1986) Diabetic Biobreeding/Worcester (BB/Wor) rats need not to be lymphopenic. J Immunol 136: 3254–3258
Lorenz RG, Allen P (1988) Direct evidence for functional self-protein/la-molecule complexes in vivo. Proc Natl Acad Sci USA 85: 5220–5223
Massa PT, TerMeulen V, Fontana A (1987) Hyperinducibility of la antigen on astrocytes correlates with satrain-specific susceptibility to experimental allergic encephalomyelitis. Proc Natl Acad Sci USA 84: 4219–4223
Miller BJ, Appel MC, O'Neill JJ, Wicker LS (1988) Both the Lyt-2 + and L3T4 + T-cell subsets are required for the transfer of diabetes in nonobese diabetic mice. J Immunol 140: 52–58
Moeller G (ed) (1985) Molecular genetics of class I and II MHC antigens. Immunol Rev 84 and 85
Mordes JP, Gallina DL, Handler ES, Greiner DL, Nakamura N, Pelletier A, Rossini AA (1987) Transfusions enriched for W3/25 + helper/inducer T lymphocytes prevent spontaneous diabetes in the BB/W rat. Diabetologia 30: 22–26
Morel PA, Dorman JS, Todd JA, McDevitt HO, Trucco M (1988) Aspartic acid at position 57 of the HLA-DQ β chain protects against type I diabetes: a family story. Proc Natl Acad Sci USA 85: 8111–8115
Mueller U, Jongeneel CV, Nedospasov SA, Fisher Lindahl K, Steinmetz M (1987) Tumor necrosis factor lymphotoxin genes map close to H-2D in the mouse major histocompatibility complex. Nature 325: 265–267
Naparstek Y, Baur K, Reis MD, Breitman L, Mak TW, Schwartz RS, Madaio MP (1988) Autoreactive T cells with a typical MHC restiction for MLR-1pr/1pr mice: forbidden clones revisited J Mol Cell Immunol 4: 35–43
Nishimoto H, Kikutani H, Yamamura KI, Kishimoto T (1987) Prevention of autoimmune insulitis by expression of I-E molecules in NOD mice. Nature 328: 432–434
Parsitol HS, Hirsch RL, Haley AS, Johnson KP (1986) Exacerbations of multiple sclerosis in patients treated with gamma interferon. Lancet 1: 893–894
Prochazka M, Leiter EH, Serreze DV, Coleman DL (1987) Three recessive loci required for insulin-dependent diabetes in nonobese diabetic mice. Science 237: 286–289
Pujol-Borrell R, Todd, Doslin M, Botazzo GF, Sutton R, Gray D, Adolf GR, Feldmann M (1987) HLA class II induction tumor islet cells by interferon-γ plus tumor necrosis factor or lymphotoxin. Nature 326: 304–307
Rossini AA, Mordes JP, Like AA (1985) Immunology of insulin-dependent diabetes mellitus. Annu Rev Immunol 3: 289
Rotter JI, Landau EM (1984) Measuring the genetic contribution of a single locus to a multilocus disease. Clin Genet 26: 529–542
Segiescu D, Cerutti I, Efthymiou E, Kahan A, Chany C (1979) Adverse effects of interferon treatment on the life span of NZB mice. Biomed Exp 31: 48

Serreze DV, Leiter E (1988) Defective activation of T suppressor cell function in nonobese diabetic mice. Potential relation to cytokine deficiencies. J Immunol 140: 3801–3807

Shizuru JA, Taylor-Edwards C, Banks BA, Gregory AK, Fathman CG (1988) Immunotherapy of the nonobese diabetic mouse: treatment with an antibody to T-helper lymphocytes. Science 240: 659–662

Todd JA, Bell JI, McDevitt HO (1987) HLA-DQ_β gene contributes to susceptibility and resistance to insulin-dependant diabetes mellitus. Nature 329: 599–604

Todd JA, Acha-Orbea H, Bell JI, Chao N, Fronek Z, Jacob CO, McDermott M, Sinha AA, Timmerman L, Steinman L, McDevitt HO (1988) A molecular basis for MHC class II-associated autoimmunity. Science 240: 1003–1009

Todd JA, Mijovic C, Fletcher J, Jenkins D, Bradwell AR, Barnett AH (1989) Identification of susceptibility loci for insulin-dependent diabetes mellitus by trans-racial gene mapping. Nature 338: 587–589

Unanue ER, Allen PM (1987) The basis for the immunoregulatory role of macrophages and other accessory cells. Science 236: 551–557

Wicker LS, Miller BJ (1988) The MHC-linked gene in the NOD mouse is not absolutely recessive. Diabetes 37: 10A

Wicker LS, Miller BJ, Coker LZ, McNally SE, Scott S, Mullen Y, Appel MC (1987) Genetic control of diabetes and insulitis in the nonobese diabetic (NOD) mouse. J Exp Med 165: 1639–1654

Woda BA, Biron CA (1986) Natural killer cell number and function in the spontaneously diabetic BB/W rat. J Immunol 137: 1860–1866

Zinkernagel RM, Dohertly PC (1979) MHC-restricted cytotoxic T cells: studies on the biological role of polymorphic major transplantation antigens determining T-cell restriction specificity, function and responsiveness. Adv Immunol 27: 52–177

Major Histocompatibility Complex Molecules and the Beta Cell: Inferences from Transgenic Models*

J. ALLISON, L. C. HARRISON, I. L. CAMPBELL, and J. F. A. P. MILLER

1 Introduction

Type 1 or insulin-dependent diabetes mellitus is a syndrome of chronic hyperglycaemia secondary to insulin deficiency due to the selective destruction of the pancreatic islet β cells. The molecular pathology of the disease in humans is still poorly understood, but a substantial body of evidence favours the view that the β cells are destroyed by an autoimmune process initiated in genetically predisposed individuals by environmental agents such as viruses or chemotoxins (EISENBARTH 1986; ROSSINI et al. 1988; CAMPBELL and HARRISON 1989). Evidence in humans for the autoimmune basis of type 1 diabetes includes the following: (a) the presence of circulating autoantibodies to islet cells and/or insulin in the majority of newly diagnosed patients (GLEICHMANN and BOTTAZZO 1987), (b) mononuclear cell infiltration or "insulitis" of islets seen in the pancreas obtained at autopsy from newly diagnosed subjects (GEPTS and LE COMPTE 1981; FOULIS et al. 1986), (c) recurrence of diabetes associated with insulitis in recipients of pancreas isografts from major histocompatibility complex (MHC) identical siblings (SIBLEY et al. 1985) and (d) an increase in the frequency and duration of remissions from insulin dependence in newly diagnosed patients treated with immunosuppressive agents (HARRISON et al. 1985; ASSAN et al. 1985).

Stronger and more direct evidence for autoimmune mechanisms in type 1 diabetes has been obtained in several natural animal models, notably the Biobreeding (BB) rat (reviewed by MARLISS et al. 1983) and the non-obese diabetic (NOD) mouse (reviewed by LEITER et al. 1987). Diabetes in these animals is associated with insulitis and is prevented by monoclonal antibodies against a number of immune effector molecules, including CD4 and CD8 molecules on T lymphocytes (LIKE et al. 1986; BENDALAC et al. 1987); furthermore, lymphocytes transferred from diabetic animals induce insulitis and diabetes in non-diabetes prone animals (KOEVARY et al. 1983; WICKER et al. 1986).

The Walter and Eliza Hall Institute of Medical Research, Parkville, Victoria 3050, Australia
* The authors are supported by the National Health and Medical Research Council of Australia and grants from Apex-Diabetes Australia, the Juvenile Diabetes Foundation and the Kellion Foundation

Current Topics in Microbiology and Immunology, Vol. 156

The onset of symptoms, which marks the clinical diagnosis of type 1 diabetes, is usually acute, reflecting the near-total lack of insulin secretory function. However, evidence from family studies (GORSUCH et al. 1981; SRIKANTA et al. 1985; TARN et al. 1987) suggests that the clinical onset is the culmination of progressive β cell destruction extending over months to years. This pre-clinical stage in humans holds the key to understanding the pathogenetic mechanisms of type 1 diabetes and developing intervention strategies for the prevention and cure of the disease (HARRISON and KAY 1989). By analogy with the natural animal models it is likely that the molecular pathology of β cell destruction in humans progresses through a number of defineable stages (HARRISON et al. 1989; CAMPBELL and HARRISON 1989). Studies in the animal models and limited post-mortem data in humans (FOULIS 1986, 1987a, b) indicate important roles for MHC molecules in the initiation of β cell destruction and its progress through these stages. This review focusses on these roles of the MHC molecules and, in particular, on the inferences from new models of type 1 diabetes in which MHC molecules have been expressed transgenically in the β cells of mice.

2 MHC Molecules and Beta Cell Pathology

Although the opportunities to study the pancreas in humans with type 1 diabetes are obviously limited, analysis of post-mortem (BOTTAZZO et al. 1985) and pancreas isograft biopsy (SIBLEY et al. 1985) specimens reveals, as in the animal models, insulitis in which $CD8^+$ T lymphocytes predominate. In addition, FOULIS et al. (1987a, b) found that human post-mortem specimens exhibited overexpression of MHC class I molecules on islet cells and aberrant expression of MHC class II molecules on β cells, in association with immunoreactive interferon-α. These changes were restricted to islets with insulin-containing cells and were often present in the absence of an inflammatory infiltrate, suggesting that they might be an early event preceding insulitis and therefore independent of cytokine production from mononuclear cells. Furthermore, the fact that overexpression of class I molecules was not always accompanied by expression of class II molecules on β cells in the same islet suggests that overexpression of class I molecules might be the primary response to whatever factor initiated the islet lesion. Whether these changes in MHC molecules are a non-specific response to injury as seen in a variety of cells after DNA damage inflicted by chemicals or UV irradiation (LAMBERT et al. 1989) or a specific response, for example to a persisting virus infection, remains to be determined.

The presence of immunoreactive interferon-α in the islets (FOULIS et al. 1987b) provides an explanation for overexpression of class I molecules in response to virus infection. Indeed, interferon-α has been shown to upregulate class I molecules in islet cells in vitro (PUJOL-BORRELL et al. 1986). One of the consequences of direct infection of cultured murine or human islet cells by reoviruses (CAMPBELL et al. 1988a), Western Nile virus or coxsackieviruses (I.L. CAMPBELL et al., unpublished) is the upregulation of class I molecules. In a rat insulinoma cell line (RINm5F), reovirus induced upregulation of mRNA for MHC class I together with mRNA for the interferon-inducible enzyme 2′,5′-oligoadenylate synthetase, but this effect was independent of new protein synthesis and detectable interferon or other soluble mediator, suggesting that the double-stranded RNA virus might directly activate the transcription of MHC class I genes (I.L. CAMPBELL et al., unpublished).

The mechanisms involved in the induction of MHC class II molecules in β cells are unknown. Although class II molecules can be induced on human β cells in vitro by the combination of interferon-γ (IFN-γ) and tumor necrosis factor (TNF) (PUJOL-BORRELL 1987; CAMPBELL et al. 1988b), these cytokines are unlikely to account for the appearance of class II molecules at the earliest stage of the islet lesion when, according to the observations of FOULIS et al. (1987a), immunoinflammatory cells are absent. On the other hand, viruses have been shown to induce class II molecules in other cell types, e.g. astrocytes (MASSA et al. 1986) and thyrocytes (NEUFELD et al. 1989).

One of the earliest changes in the islets in the animal models of type 1 diabetes that accompanies hyperexpression of class I molecules is the appearance of activated macrophages (KOLB-BACHOFEN and KOLB 1989). The antigen(s) to which these macrophages are responding has not been identified. That β cells in the islet lesion can sometimes express class II molecules led to the hypothesis that aberrant expression of class II molecules might allow β cells to present autoantigens directly to T lymphocytes and thereby initiate autoimmunity (BOTTAZZO et al. 1983). However, effective antigen presentation and T lymphocyte activation is a multifactorial process requiring adhesion of T lymphocytes to antigen-presenting cells (reviewed by WARWRYK et al. 1989), interaction of the T-cell receptor with the MHC class II molecule bearing processed antigen peptide (UNANUE and ALLEN 1987), production by the antigen-presenting cell of primary T lymphocyte growth and differentiation factors termed co-stimulators, e.g. interleukin-1 or interleukin-6 (GARMAN et al. 1987; LOTZ et al. 1988) and possibly the interaction of other accessory molecules on both the antigen-presenting cell and the T lymphocyte. Therefore, it is unlikely that the "aberrant" expression of class II molecules alone would be sufficient to permit the β cell to be its own antigen-presenting cell. Experiments in mice transgenically expressing class II molecules, discussed below, directly support this idea.

Activated mononuclear cells infiltrating the islets early in the development of insulitis would be a source of cytokines, two of which, IFN-γ and TNF, significantly impair β cell function and morphology (CAMPBELL et al. 1988c) and, potentially, enhance islet cell immunoreactivity by upregulating the expression of class I molecules and inducing the expression of class II molecules on islet cells (CAMPBELL et al. 1985, 1988b; PUJOL-BORRELL et al. 1987). Although these changes in the expression of MHC molecules may not, in themselves, be sufficient for activation of autoreactive T lymphocytes, they could certainly enhance the response of T lymphocytes pre-activated to β cell antigens presented on classical antigen-presenting cells. On the other hand, other effects of cytokines might confer on the β cell the properties of a classical antigen-presenting cell. Thus, IFN-γ or TNF-α induce the expression of the intercellular adhesion molecule ICAM-1 on human islet cells (CAMPBELL et al. 1989a) and at the same time also induce islet cells to secrete IL-6 (CAMPBELL et al. 1989b), which is a co-stimulator for T lymphocytes (GARMAN et al. 1987; LOTZ et al. 1988). Together with the hyperexpression of class I molecules and the induction of class II molecules, the induction of ICAM-1 expression and IL-6 secretion by islet cells may be sufficient to permit them to present antigen and perpetuate their own destruction (CAMPBELL and HARRISON 1989). The specificity of the process for β cells within the islet presumably reflects the presence of a β cell-specific antigen and/or a differential sensitivity of β cells to the effects of cytokines and other mediators. In the presence of β cell-specific autoantigens cytokines could be delivered in a targeted fashion into the micro-environment of the β cell or even directly into the β cell by adherent cytotoxic T lymphocytes. Concomitant upregulation of class I molecules would enhance the targeting of cytotoxic T lymphocytes.

3 Hyperexpression of MHC Molecules—A Common Denominator of β Cell Dysfunction?

As already discussed, overexpression of class I molecules is an early feature of the islet lesion of type 1 diabetes in humans and animal models and is a concomitant of impaired β cell function in response to certain viruses and cytokines. It may also be relevant that we have observed increased expression of class I molecules on human insulinoma cells (OXBROW et al. 1988) and on relatively undifferentiated rat insulinoma cells (R. BARTHOLOMEUSZ et al., unpublished), implying that there may be an inverse relationship between class I expression and differentiated function is β cells. These observations suggested to us that overexpression of class I molecules might not only enhance immune responses, but have a direct, non-immune effect to impair β cell function (HARRISON et al. 1989). Transgenic mouse models provide a means of examining this question by enabling MHC genes to be overexpressed in β cells from an early stage in development.

4 Transgenic Mouse Models

Transgenic mice are created by injecting purified DNA into the nucleus of fertilized mouse eggs and reimplanting these eggs into the oviduct of pseudopregnant female mice (BRINSTER et al. 1985). The eggs that develop may incorporate the DNA into one, or rarely, two sites of the mouse chromosomes. This integration event is generally random and accompanied by a tandem duplication of the new DNA so that between one and several hundred copies of the DNA come to reside at a chromosome locus. If the integration takes place in one cell of a cleavage embryo, rather than in the single cell egg, the resulting transgenic founder mouse may be mosaic; that is, only a proportion of its somatic or germ cell tissues will carry the transgene (WILKIE et al. 1986). By mating the founder with non-transgenic mice the transgene will be passed on to some of the offspring which will carry it in every cell. The Mendelian inheritance of the new locus is usually stable from generation to generation, although, when searched for, rearrangements of the tandem array have been reported (PALMITER et al. 1982; PALMITER 1986).

The developmental and tissue-specific expression of the new gene will depend on the presence of the gene regulatory elements that are associated with it. The insulin gene is expressed in the β cells of the pancreatic islets and this pattern of expression is mediated by DNA sequences that lie just upstream from the sequences that actually code for the insulin pro-protein (WALKER et al. 1983). Hanahan has shown that the rat insulin upstream element can direct the expression of other protein coding sequences, for example the SV40 T antigen, to the islet β cells of transgenic mice (HANAHAN 1985). This transgene expression closely parallels that of the endogenous mouse insulin gene, but differs slightly in onset and in the levels of protein (ALPERT et al. 1988). Furthermore, transgenes composed of regulatory elements from different genes often show entirely unexpected patterns of gene expression. For example, the rat insulin promoter directs the expression of class II MHC molecules to the islet β cells, but the combination of this element and the class II genomic sequences results in novel expression in the kidney tubule epithelium (LO et al. 1988).

4.1 Class I β Cell Transgenic Mice

A number of experiments have used the transgenic mouse system to test the relevance to diabetes of MHC expression in the β cells (Table 1). ALLISON et al. (1988) introduced the class I H-2K^b gene linked to the rat insulin II promoter into the germline of mouse strains that were syngeneic or allogeneic with respect to the transgene product. This resulted in the abundant expression of H-2K^b heavy chain protein in the islet β cells which normally express only very low levels of class I molecules (BAEKKESKOV et al. 1981). It was expected that when the K^b product was present as non-self it would provoke an immune response. However, the B10 congenic founder mice that were syngeneic (haplotype bk) or allogeneic (haplotype kk) with respect to the transgene all developed diabetes from an early age. Three (C57BL/6 × SJL)F2 founder mice of haplotypes bs, bb and ss were normal, but their transgenic offspring were all diabetic regardless of haplotype. These founder mice were therefore mosaics and had sufficient numbers of non-transgenic β cells to maintain normal blood glucose levels. Differences in the severity of the diabetes were seen in different mouse strains, B10.BR being

Table 1. Transgenes expressed in mouse pancreatic β cells

Regulatory element	Transgene product	Diabetes	Refere[illegible]
Rat insulin II	Class I MHC: H-2K^b	Yes	Allis[illegible]t al. (1988)
Human insulin	Class II MHC: I-Aα^d/Aβ^d	Yes	Sarvetnick et al. (1988)
Rat insulin II	Class II MHC: I-E$^d_\alpha$E$^b_\beta$ (I-E^b)	Yes	Lo et al. (1988)
Rat insulin II	Class II MHC: I-A^k	No	D. Mathis (personal communication)
Rat insulin II	Influenza haemagglutinin	Disruption of islet architecture. Most mice hyperglycaemic but only a minority overtly diabetic	J. Sambrook (personal communication)
Human insulin	Herpes simplex glycoprotein D	No	T. Stewart (personal communication)
Human insulin	Human insulin	Impairment of mouse insulin secretion	D. Steiner (personal communication)
Rat insulin II	Chicken calmodulin	Yes	P.C. Epstein (personal communication)
Human insulin	Mouse interferon-γ	Yes	Savetnick et al. (1988)
Rat insulin II	Oncogenes		
	SV40 T antigen	No	
	H-*ras*	Yes (males only)	
	Human p53	No	
	Mouse p53	No	Adams et al. (1987)
	Mouse *c-myc*	No	D.C. Hanahan (personal communication)
	Mouse *v-fos*	No	
	Human placental lactogen	No	
	Polyoma large T antigen	No	
	Polyoma middle T antigen	No	

particularly susceptible and incapable of breeding. The disease was identified as type 1 diabetes because of persistent glucosuria and weight loss that could be controlled by daily insulin injections. In addition, total pancreatic insulin content (Fig. 1) and islet number (Table 2) were significantly reduced.

The occurrence of diabetes in strains of mice syngeneic with respect to the K^b transgene product was unexpected and suggested that the hyperexpression of class I heavy chain molecules in the β cells might alone be responsible for the disease. Histology of the newly diabetic pancreas showed abnormal islets depleted of β cells, but still containing the glucagon-producing α cells and the somatostatin producing δ cells. The α and δ cells persisted, while all the β cells were lost by about 50 days after the onset of diabetes. Most importantly, no lymphocytic infiltrate was detected in the islets at any time after birth. The

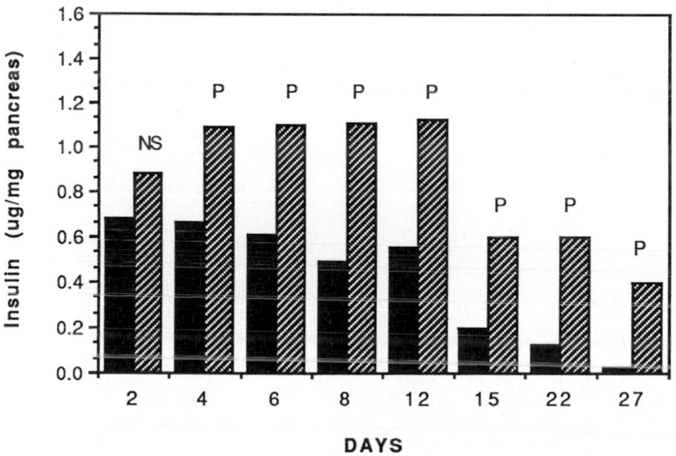

Fig. 1. Insulin content of pancreas from transgenic (*solid bars*) and non-transgenic (*hatched bars*) mice. *NS*, not significant; $P < 0.001$

Table 2. Islet isolation from 14-day transgenic and non-transgenic mice

Mouse	Fasting blood glucose (mM)	Islets: Yield	Islets: Appearance	Transgenic
1	2.4	55	++	—
2	2.9	119	+++	—
3	2.5	80	+++	—
4	3.1	74	+++	—
5	3.9	15	+	+
6	4.4	38	+	+
7	4.5	70	++	+
8	3.3	42	+	+

+++ normal contrast; ++ low contrast; + very low contrast on black background

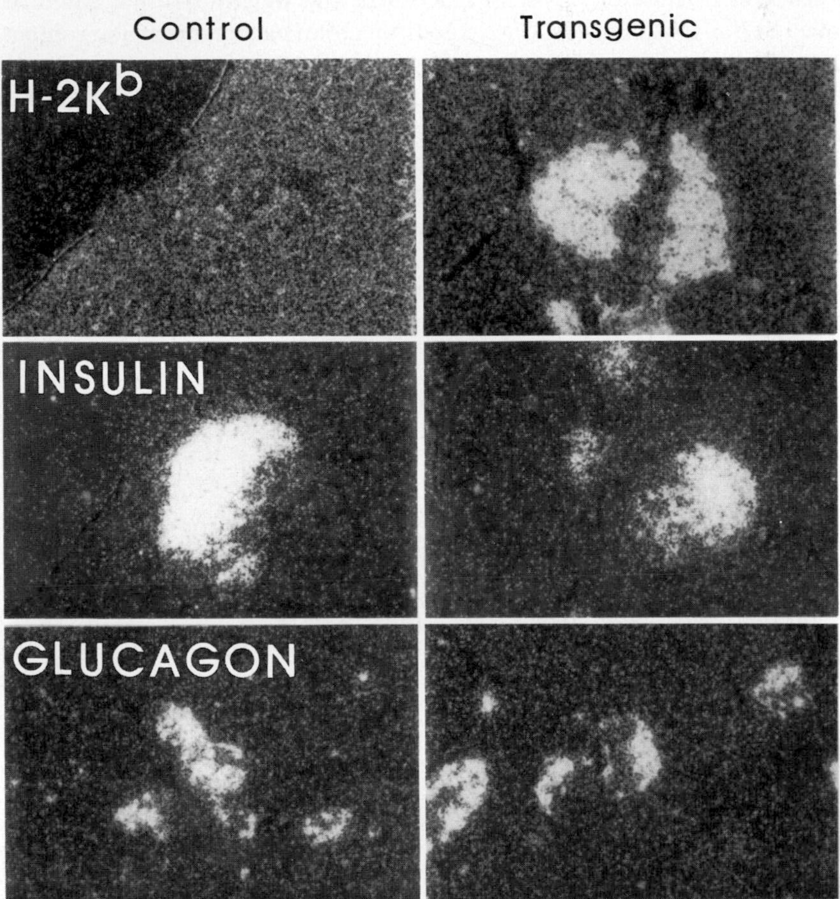

Fig. 2. In situ hybridization of mouse class I MHC (H-2K^b) and rat glucagon cDNA probes (labelled with ^{35}S-α-ATP), and an oligonucleotide (30-mer) to the rat insulin sequence (end-labelled with ^{32}P-γ-ATP), to 6 μm frozen sections of control and H-2K^b transgenic mouse pancreas. The expression of insulin mRNA was reproducibly decreased in transgenic compared to control islets at day 14, but not apparently to the same extent as insulin protein content and secretion (L.C. HARRISON et al., unpublished)

expression of the K^b protein in the β cells was observed by immunocytochemistry using monoclonal antibodies specific for K^b and by in situ hybridization (Fig. 2). The K^b protein was expressed at day 16 in the transgenic embryo and was present until all the β cells were lost. However, the staining pattern was predominantly cytoplasmic, as expected, because the class I heavy chain requires β-2 microglobulin to be transported to the cell surface (SEVERINSSON and PETERSON 1984).

The level of K^b surface expression was low, as demonstrated by flow cytometric analysis. For high level surface expression of the transgenic class I protein, mice may have to be made transgenic for both the K^b heavy chain and β-2 microglobulin under the influence of the rat insulin promoter.

Confirmation of the non-immune involvement of the class I K^b molecules in the diabetes process was obtained by comparing insulin secretion from transgenic and non-transgenic fetal pancreata cultured in vitro for 18 days (T. MANDEL, personal communication). Transgenic fetal pancreata had impaired secretion of insulin over a time course that paralleled the decrease in insulin content of pancreata isolated from mice at equivalent ages (Fig. 1). In addition, backcrossing the K^b transgene onto C57BL/6 nude mice still resulted in diabetes, demonstrating that β cell destruction occurred in systems in which no immune cells were present.

4.2 Class II β Cell Transgenic Mice

Islet β cells do not normally express class II MHC molecules. Two groups have introduced class II genes into transgenic mice to test whether the presence of class II proteins on the β cell surface is sufficient to induce autoimmunity by presenting islet antigens to T cells (Table 1). SARVETNICK et al. (1988) chose the I-A molecule and LO et al. (1988) used an I-E molecule. In the case of I-A β cell transgenics the human insulin promoter was used to direct the separate expression of the I-Aα^d and I-Aβ^d genes to islet β cells of H-2^d mice. Expression of either the α or β chain alone failed to induce diabetes. However, when Ins-I-A α and Ins-I-A β transgenics were mated, only those offspring that carried both I-A chains became diabetic. For Ins-I-E transgenics the rat insulin promoter was used to direct the expression of the I-Eα^d and I-Eβ^b genes to β cells of mouse strains that lacked endogenous I-E or had the same I-E haplotype as the transgene. All mice expressing the I-E molecules in the β cells became diabetic. Interestingly, these mice also expressed transgenic I-E molecules in the kidney tubule epithelium, which is known not to be a site of expression of class II molecules. The pattern of disease for the β cell class II transgenics was very similar to that described for the class I transgenics above, and no autoimmune reaction was seen in the islets of these Ins-I-A or Ins-I-E mice, or in the kidney of the Ins-I-E mice.

One further experiment using class II β cell transgenics failed to support the previous findings. MATHIS et al. (D. MATHIS, personal communication) bred class II I-A^k transgenic mice using cDNA coding sequences and the rat insulin promoter (Table 1). These mice expressed lower levels of class II in the β cells than found in the Ins-I-E or Ins-I-A^d mice and did not become diabetic. It is possible that a critical level of expression is required for diabetes to occur. A comparison between the different class II β cell transgenics may help define this level of expression.

5 Relevance of MHC β Cell Transgenics to Diabetes

The non-immune destruction of β cells by overexpression of MHC molecules in transgenic mice is a significant finding in light of the strong evidence for autoimmune-mediated type 1 diabetes. It is important therefore to consider how relevant a transgenic mouse system is to the other models of diabetes and to human type I diabetes itself. Is the transgenic model merely an artefact resulting from greatly over-expressed levels of RNA or protein in the β cells? Firstly, do the additional copies of the transgene promoter compete for factors necessary for transcription of the mouse insulin gene itself? This is not supported by the observation that in the Ins-I-A β cell transgenics both α and β chain expression is required for diabetes to occur; presence of one of the chains results in abundant RNA transcription, but no diabetes (SARVETNICK et al. 1988). The mild hyperglycaemia associated with Ins-I-Aα transgenics may result from slight upregulation of the endogenous I-Eβ chain in the β cells, creating a functional chimeric class II molecule (SARVETNICK et al. 1988). Secondly, could the over-expression of any protein result in competition with insulin for factors necessary for protein synthesis, processing or transport? A number of secretory and membrane-bound proteins have been over-expressed in islet β cells with no deleterious effects (Table 1). However, the H-*ras* oncogene and the influenza haemagglutinin protein did result in limited β cell dysfunction (Table 1). The pathology of islet death by transgenic MHC molecules closely resembles that in other models of diabetes except for the lack of insulitis. Furthermore, it is remarkably like that seen in the islets of humans with diabetes who died before 18 months of age, where no insulitis but overexpression of MHC molecules was observed (FOULIS et al. 1986). On the other hand, the transgenic overexpression of H-*ras* and influenza haemagglutinin resulted in a most unusual pathology with large holes in the centre of the islets. This pattern of destruction has not been reported in any of the known models of diabetes. It is, at present, difficult to determine absolutely the specificity of MHC molecules in islet cell destruction. However, it is quite reasonable to consider that the overexpression of MHC molecules seen in islets in animal models and in human type 1 diabetes might contribute to the destruction of β cells by a non-immune mechanism.

6 Mechanisms of β Cell Destruction by MHC Molecules

The problem of how overexpression of MHC molecules might lead to β cell death is difficult to address. It may simply interfere non-specifically with the insulin secretory pathway, as discussed above. However, in the class I β cell transgenics the expression of class I K^b molecules in the β cells is only a fraction of that of insulin protein. A defect at the level of insulin secretion is suggested by the data on the total pancreas insulin content (Fig. 1). Although the class I MHC mice are severely diabetic at 18 days of age, their insulin content is only fourfold lower than non-transgenic controls. Indeed, glucose-stimulated insulin release from the islets of transgenic mice, ex vivo, is defective, indicating that the insulin present in the β cells of diabetic transgenics is not released into the blood (ALLISON et al. 1988). Discussion on why insulin secretion is defective can only be speculative. MHC molecules bind peptides (BJORKMAN et al. 1987) and have been reported to interact non-covalently with several membrane receptors (SIMONSEN et al. 1985) and with an adenovirus glycoprotein in the endoplasmic reticulum (ANDERSSON et al. 1985). The class I or class II molecules may interact with proinsulin or insulin at some point in the secretory pathway or with other molecules such as receptors whose function is critical for normal cell function. Perhaps the association of a protein destined for the membrane with one destined for secretion prevents the normal processing of insulin, as discussed by PARHAM (1988).

7 β Cell Transgenics as a Model of Tolerance

The lack of an immune response to foreign MHC molecules expressed in the islet β cells defied prediction. Possibly, the very early onset of expression, before immunocompetent T cells have developed, allows tolerance to occur (BILLINGHAM et al. 1953). In contrast, late onset expression might lead to an immune response analogous to that in RIP-SV40 transgenics (ADAMS et al. 1987). In this latter model, expression of SV40 T antigen in β cells before birth led to tolerance, whereas expression some weeks after birth resulted in an immune response to the β cells expressing the T antigen. However, MARKMANN et al. (1988) have shown that fetal islets expressing transgenic I-E molecules did not provoke an immune reaction when they were transplanted into normal I-E negative adult mice. Hence, late presentation of β cell I-E to T cells is not a requirement for immune reactivity. A reaction was seen only if the host mice were primed against the I-E antigen by injecting I-E antigen-presenting cells from the spleen and concomitantly transplanting transgenic-I-E fetal islets. This indicates a requirement by the host T cells for an activating "second signal" which the β cells are normally unable to provide (LAFFERTY 1980). These findings may explain the results of SARVETNICK et al. (1988) who found massive insulitis and autoimmunity when IFN-γ was overexpressed in the β cells. This resulted in upregulation of class II MHC (class I overexpression was not investigated) in the islets and acinar tissue. IFN-γ would also presumably induce the expression of ICAM-1 and the secretion of IL-6, as demonstrated in vitro (CAMPBELL et al. 1989a, b), and perhaps provide the signals needed to activate T cells to recognize islet cell or acinar cell antigen presented to them by the upregulated class II molecules (CAMPBELL and HARRISON 1989).

In class I β cell transgenics, the continued presence of allogeneic MHC antigen in the β cell was required to maintain T cell tolerance in vitro (MORAHAN et al. 1989). Peripheral T cells isolated from transgenics at an early age did not react to the transgene MHC molecules in an in vitro cytotoxic T lymphocyte assay, but gave a response when isolated from old transgenics which had lost their β cells and, hence, the allogeneic MHC molecules. This suggests that tolerance is actively maintained by a peripheral mechanism, but does not explain how the tolerizing process occurs. Thymic lymphocytes of the young class I β cell transgenics were not tolerant in vitro, suggesting that tolerance does not result from shed allo-antigen circulating back to the thymus and imposing clonal deletion on potentially reactive thymus lymphocytes. Possibly, functional silencing of T cells, i.e. T cell anergy, takes place in the absence of a second signal which, as mentioned above, the β cell cannot normally provide. Evidence for this comes from the work of MARKMANN et al. (1988) who showed that isolated Ins-I-E β cells were able to tolerize T cell lines in vitro.

The MHC transgenic experiments demonstrate that class I or class II expression in the β cells is alone not sufficient to confer antigen-presenting function on the β cells and is therefore unlikely to initiate autoimmunity. This result is apparently contradictory to the hypothesis of BOTTAZZO et al. (1983) that "aberrant" expression of class II MHC by endocrine epithelial cells triggers autoimmunity. Nevertheless, T cells already activated against class II molecules could recognize them on β cells (MARKMANN et al. 1988). We have proposed that the induction of class II molecules in the β cell is a necessary, but not sufficient step for antigen presentation and that effective "phenotypic switching" of the β cell for the role of antigen presentation also requires induction and expression of ICAM-1, and possibly other adhesion molecules, and secretion of IL-6 as co-stimulator (CAMPBELL and HARRISON 1989). The transgenic experiments demonstrate, however, that the overexpression of MHC molecules can have a direct, non-immune detrimental effect on β cells which in vivo, e.g., in response to virus infection, could be the early pre-autoimmune lesion.

Acknowledgements. The technical assistance of Adrienne Wilson and the secretarial assistance of Joyce Lygnos are greatly appreciated.

References

Adams TE, Alpert S, Hanahan D (1987) Non-tolerance and autoantibodies to a transgenic self antigen expressed in pancreatic β cells. Nature 325: 223–228

Allison J, Campbell IL, Morahan G, Mandel TE, Harrison LC, Miller JFAP (1988) Diabetes in transgenic mice resulting from over-expression of class I histocompatibility molecules in pancreatic β cells. Nature 333: 529–533

Alpert S, Hanahan D, Teitelman G (1988) Hybrid insulin genes reveal a developmental lineage for pancreatic endocrine cells and imply a relationship with neurons. Cell 53: 295–308

Andersson M, Pääbo S, Nilsson T, Peterson P (1985) Impaired intracellular transport of class I MHC antigens as a possible means for adnenovirus to evade immune surveillance. Cell 43: 215–222
Assan R, Feutren G, Debray-Sachs M, Quiniou-Debrie MC, Laborie C, Thomas G, Chatenoud L, Bach JF (1985) Metabolic and immunological effects of cyclosporin in recently diagnosed type 1 diabetes mellitus. Lancet 1: 67–71
Baekkeskov S, Kanatsuna T, Klareskog L, Nielsen DA, Peterson A, Rubenstein AH, Steiner DF, Lernmark A (1981) Expression of major histocompatibility antigens on pancreatic islet cells. Proc Natl Acad Sci USA 78: 6456–6460
Bendelac A, Carnaud C, Boitard C, Bach JF (1987) Syngeneic transfer of autoimmune diabetes from diabetic NOD mice to healthy neonates. Requirement for both L3T4$^+$ and Lyt-2$^+$ T cells. J Exp Med 166: 823–832
Billingham RE, Breur L, Medawar PB (1953) "Actively acquired tolerance" of foreign cells. Nature 172: 603–606
Bjorkman PJ, Saper MA, Samraoui B, Bennett WS, Strominger JL, Wiley DC (1987) The foreign antigen binding site and T cell recognition regions of class I histocompatibility antigens. Nature 329: 512–518
Bottazzo GF, Pujol-Borrell R, Hanafusa T, Feldmann M (1983) Hypothesis: role of aberrant HLA-DR expression and antigen presentation in the induction of endocrine autoimmunity. Lancet 2: 1115
Bottazzo GF, Dean BM, McNally JM, Mackay EH, Swift PGF, Gamble DR (1985) In situ characterization of autoimmune phenomena and expression of HLA molecules in the pancreas in diabetic insulitis. N Engl J Med 31: 353–360
Brinster RL, Chen HY, Trumbauer ME, Yagle MK, Palmiter RD (1985) Factors affecting the efficiency of introducing foreign DNA into mice by microinjecting eggs. Proc Natl Acad Sci USA 82: 4438–4442
Campbell IL, Harrison LC (1989) Molecular pathology of type 1 diabetes. Mol Biol Med (in press)
Campbell IL, Wong GHW, Schrader JW, Harrison LC (1985) Interferon-γ enhances the expression of the major histocompatibility class I antigens on mouse pancreatic beta cells. Diabetes 34: 1205–1209
Campbell IL, Harrison LC, Ashcroft RG, Jack I (1988a) Reovirus infection enhances expression of class I MHC proteins on human β-cell and rat RINm5F cell. Diabetes 37: 362–365
Campbell IL, Oxbrow L, West J, Harrison LC (1988b) Regulation of MHC protein expression in pancreatic beta cells by interferon-γ and tumor necrosis factor-α. Mol Endocrinol 2: 101–107
Campbell IL, Iscaro A, Harrison LC (1988c) Interferon-γ and tumor necrosis factor-α: cytotoxicity to murine islets of Langerhans. J Immunol 141: 2325–2329
Campbell IL, Cutri A, Wilkinson D, Boyd AW, Harrison LC (1989a) Intercellular adhesion molecule-1 is induced on endocrine islet cells by cytokines but not by reovirus infection. Proc Natl Acad Sci USA 86: 4282–4286
Campbell IL, Cutri A, Wilson A, Harrison LC (1989b) Evidence of interleukin-6 production by and effects on the pancreatic beta cell. J Immunol 143: 1188–1191
Eisenbarth GS (1986) Type 1 diabetes mellitus. A chronic autoimmune disease. N Engl J Med 314: 1360–1368
Foulis AK, Liddle CN, Farquharson MA, Richmond JA (1986) The histopathology of the pancreas in type 1 (insulin-dependent) diabetes mellitus: a 25-year review of deaths in patients under 20 years of age in the United Kingdom. Diabetologia 29: 267–274
Foulis AK, Farquharson MA, Hardman R (1987a) Aberrant expression of class II major histocompatibility complex molecules by β cells and hyperexpression of class I major histocompatibility complex molecules by insulin containing islets in type 1 (insulin-dependent) diabetes mellitus. Diabetologia 30: 333–343
Foulis AK, Farquharson MA, Meager A (1987b) Immunoreactive alpha-interferon in insulin-secreting beta cells in type 1 diabetes mellitus. Lancet 2: 1423–1427
Garman RD, Jacobs KA, Clark SC, Raulet DH (1987) B-cell stimulating factor 2 (β2 interferon) functions as a second signal for interleukin-2 production by mature murine T cells. Proc Natl Acad Sci USA 84: 7629–7633
Gepts W, Lecompte PM (1981) The pancreatic islets in diabetes. Am J Med 70: 105–115
Gleichman H, Bottazzo GF (1987) Islet cell and insulin autoantibodies in diabetes. Immunol Today 8: 167–168
Gorsuch AN, Lister J, Dean BM, Spencer KM, NcNally JM, Bottazzo GF, Cudworth AG (1981) Evidence for a long prediabetic period in type 1 (insulin-dependent) diabetes mellitus. Lancet 2: 1363–1365

Hanahan D (1985) Heritable formation of pancreatic β-cell tumours in transgenic mice expressing recombinant insulin/simian virus 40 oncogenes. Nature 315: 115–122

Harrison LC, Kay TWH (1989) Strategies for intervention therapy in type 1 diabetes. In: Andreani D, Kolb H, Pozzilli P (eds) Immunotherapy of type 1 diabetes. Wiley, Chichester, pp 93–110

Harrison LC, Colman PG, Dean B, Baxter R, Martin FIR (1985) Increase in remission rate in newly diagnosed type 1 diabetic subjects treated with azathioprine. Diabetes 34: 1306–1308

Harrison LC, Campbell IL, Allison J, Miller JFAP (1989) MHC molecules and beta cell destruction: immune and non-immune mechanisms. Diabetes 38: 815–818

Koevary S, Rossini A, Stoller W, Chick W, Williams RM (1983) Passive transfer of diabetes in the BB/W rat. Science 220: 727–728

Kolb-Bachofen V, Kolb H (1989) A role for macrophages in the pathogenesis of type 1 diabetes. Autoimmunity 3: 145–155

Lafferty KJ, Andrus L, Prowse SJ (1980) Role of lymphokine and antigen in the control of specific T cell responses. Immunol Rev 51: 279–314

Lambert ME, Ronai ZA, Weinstein IB, Garrels JI (1989) Enhancement of major histocompatibility class I protein synthesis by DNA damage in cultured human fibroblasts and keratinocytes. Mol Cell Biol 9: 847–850

Leiter EH, Prochazka M, Coleman DL (1987) The non-obese diabetic (NOD) mouse. Am J Pathol 128: 380–393

Like AA, Biron CA, Weringer EJ, Byman K, Sroczynski E, Guberski DL (1986) Prevention of diabetes in BioBreeding/Worcester rats with monoclonal antibodies that recognize T lymphocytes or natural killer cells. J Exp Med 164: 1145–1159

Lo D, Burkly LC, Widera G, Cowing C, Flavell RA, Palmiter R, Brinster RL (1988) Diabetes and tolerance in transgenic mice expressing class II MHC molecules in pancreatic beta cells. Cell 53: 159–168

Lotz M, Jirik F, Kabouridis P, Tsoukas C, Hirano T, Kishimoto T, Carson DA (1988) B cell stimulating factor 2/interleukin-6 is a co-stimulant for human thyrocytes and T lymphocytes. J Exp Med 167: 1253–1258

Markmann J, Lo D, Naji A, Palmiter RD, Brinster RL, Heber-Katz E (1988) Antigen presenting function of class II MHC expressing pancreatic beta cells. Nature 336: 476–479

Marliss EB, Nakhooda AF, Poussier P (1983) Clinical forms and natural history of the diabetic syndrome and insulin and glucagon secretion in the BB rat. Metabolish 32 [Suppl 1]: 11–16

Massa PT, Dörries R, ter Meulen V (1986) Viral particles induce Ia antigen expression on astrocytes. Nature 320: 543–546

Morahan G, Allison J, Miller JFAP (1989) Tolerance of class I histocompatibility antigens expressed extrathymically. Nature 339: 622–624

Neufeld DS, Platzer M, Davies TF (1989) Reovirus induction of MHC class II antigen in rat thyroid cells. Endocrinology 124: 543–545

Oxbrow L, Campbell IL, Harrison LC (1988) Expression of islet cell differentiation antigens and major histocompatibility antigens on human insulinoma cells. Diabetes Res Clin Prac 5 [Suppl 1]: S140

Palmiter RD (1986) Germ-line transformation of mice. Annu Rev Genet 20: 465–499

Palmiter RD, Chen HY, Brinster RL (1982) Differential regulation of metallothionein-thymidine kinase fusion genes in transgenic mice and their offspring. Cell 29: 701–710

Parham P (1988) Intolerable secretion in tolerant transgenic mice. Nature 333: 500–503

Pujol-Borrell T, Todd I, Mala Doshi D, Gray M, Feldmann M, Bottazzo GF (1986) Differential expression and regulation of MHC products in the endocrine and exocrine cells of the human pancreas. Clin Exp Immunol 65: 128–139

Pujol-Borrell R, Todd I, Doshi M, Bottazzo GF, Sutton R, Gray R, Adolf GR, Feldmann M (1987) HLA class II induction in human islet cells by interferon-gamma plus tumour necrosis factor or lymphotoxin. Nature 326: 304–306

Rossini AA, Mordes JP, Handler ES (1988) Perspectives in diabetes: speculations on etiology of diabetes mellitus. Diabetes 37: 257–261

Sarvetnick N, Liggitt D, Pitts SL, Hansen SE, Stewart TA (1988) Insulin-dependent diabetes mellitus induced in transgenic mice by ectopic expression of class II MHC and interferon-gamma. Cell 52: 773–782

Severinsson L, Peterson PA (1984) β2-microglobulin induces intracellular transport of human class I transplantation antigen heavy chains in xenopus laevis oocytes. J Cell Biol 99: 226–232

Sibley RK, Sutherland DER, Goetz F, Michael AF (1985) Recurrent diabetes mellitus in the pancreas iso- and allograft. Lab Invest 53: 132–144

Simonsen M, Skjødt K, Crone M, Sanderson A, Fujita-Yamaguchi Y, Due C, Rønne E, Linnet K, Olsson L (1985) Compound receptors in the cell membrane: ruminations from the borderland of immunology and physiology. Prog Allergy 36: 151–176

Srikanta S, Granda OP, Rabizadeh A, Soeldner JS, Eisenbarth GS (1985) First-degree relatives of patients with type 1 diabetes mellitus. Islet cell antibodies and abnormal insulin secretion. N Engl J Med 313: 461–464

Tarn AC, Smith CP, Spencer KM, Bottazzo GF, Gale EAM (1987) Type 1 (insulin-dependent) diabetes: a disease of slow clinical onset? B Med J 294: 342–345

Unanue ER, Allen PM (1987) The basis for the immuno-regulatory role of macrophages and other accessory cells. Science 236: 551–559

Walker MD, Edlund T, Boulet AM, Rutter WJ (1983) Cell-specific expression controlled by the 5′ flanking region of insulin and chymotrypsin genes. Nature 306: 557–561

Wawryk SO, Novotny JR, Wicks IP, Wilkinson D, Maher D, Salvaris E, Welch K, Fecondo J, Boyd AW (1989) The role of the LFA-1/ICAM-1 interaction in human leukocyte homing and adhesion. Immunol Rev 108: 135–161

Wicker LS, Miller BJ, Muller Y (1986) Transfer of autoimmune diabetes mellitus with splenocytes from non-obese diabetic (NOD) mice. Diabetes 35: 855–860

Wilkie TM, Brinster RL, Palmiter RD (1986) Germline and somatic mosaicism in transgenic mice. Dev Biol 118: 9–18

Subject Index

Current Topics in Microbiology and Immunology

Volumes published since 1978 (and still available)

Vol. 80: 1978. 31 figs., 17 tab. IV, 169 pp. ISBN 3-540-08781-8

Vol. 89: **Weiss, D. W.:** Tumor Antigenicity and Approaches to Tumor Immunotherapy. An Outline. 1980. IX, 83 pp. ISBN 3-540-09789-9

Vol. 94/95: 1981. 46 figs. IV, 308 pp. ISBN 3-540-10803-3

Vol. 100: **Boehmer, H. V.; Haas, W.; Köhler, G.; Melchers, F.; Zeuthen, J. (Ed.):** T Cell Hybridomas. A Workshop at the Basel Institute for Immunology. With the collaboration Buser-Boyd, S. 1982. 52 figs. XI, 262 pp. ISBN 3-540-11535-8

Vol. 101: **Graf, Thomas; Jaenisch, Rudolf (Ed.):** Tumorviruses, Neoplastic Transformation, and Differentiation. 1982. 27 figs. VIII, 198 pp. ISBN 3-540-11665-6

Vol. 106: **Vogt, Peter K.; Koprowski, Hilary (Ed.):** Mouse Mammary Tumor Virus. 1983. 12 figs. VII, 103 pp. ISBN 3-540-12828-X

Vol. 107: **Vogt, Peter K.; Koprowski; Hilary (Ed.):** Retroviruses 2. 1983. 26 figs. VII, 180 pp. ISBN 3-540-12384-9

Vol. 109: **Doerfler, Walter (Ed.):** The Molecular Biology of Adenoviruses 1. 30 Years of Adenovirus Research 1953–1983. 1983. 69 figs. XII, 232 pp. ISBN 3-540-13034-9

Vol. 110: **Doerfler, Walter (Ed.):** The Molecular Biology of Adenoviruses 2. 30 Years of Adenovirus Research 1953–1983. 1984. 49 figs. VIII, 265 pp. ISBN 3-540-13127-2

Vol. 112: **Vogt, Peter K.; Koprowski, Hilary (Ed.):** Retroviruses 3. 1984. 19 figs. VII, 115 pp. ISBN 3-540-13307-0

Vol. 113: **Potter, Michael; Melchers, Fritz; Weigert, Martin (Ed.):** Oncogenes in B-Cell Neoplasia. Workshop at the National Cancer Institute, National Institutes of Health, Bethesda, MD March 5–7, 1984. 1984. 65 figs. XIII, 268 pp. ISBN 3-540-13597-9

Vol. 115: **Vogt, Peter K. (Ed.):** Human T-Cell Leukemia Virus. 1985. 74 figs. IX, 266 pp. ISBN 3-540-13963-X

Vol. 116: **Willis, Dawn B. (Ed.):** Iridoviridae. 1985. 65 figs. X, 173 pp. ISBN 3-540-15172-9

Vol. 122: **Potter, Michael (Ed.):** The BALB/c Mouse. Genetics and Immunology. 1985. 85 figs. XVI, 254 pp. ISBN 3-540-15834-0

Vol. 124: **Briles, David E. (Ed.):** Genetic Control of the Susceptibility to Bacterial Infection. 1986. 19 figs. XII, 175 pp. ISBN 3-540-16238-0

Vol. 125: **Wu, Henry C.; Tai, Phang C. (Ed.):** Protein Secretion and Export in Bacteria. 1986. 34 figs. X, 211 pp. ISBN 3-540-16593-2

Vol. 126: **Fleischer, Bernhard; Reimann, Jörg; Wagner, Hermann (Ed.):** Specificity and Function of Clonally Developing T-Cells. 1986. 60 figs. XV, 316 pp. ISBN 3-540-16501-0

Vol. 127: **Potter, Michael; Nadeau, Joseph H.; Cancro, Michael P. (Ed.):** The Wild Mouse in Immunology. 1986. 119 figs. XVI, 395 pp. ISBN 3-540-16657-2

Vol. 128: 1986. 12 figs. VII, 122 pp. ISBN 3-540-16621-1

Vol. 129: 1986. 43 figs., VII, 215 pp. ISBN 3-540-16834-6

Vol. 130: **Koprowski, Hilary; Melchers, Fritz (Ed.):** Peptides as Immunogens. 1986. 21 figs. X, 86 pp. ISBN 3-540-16892-3

Vol. 131: **Doerfler, Walter; Böhm, Petra (Ed.):** The Molecular Biology of Baculoviruses. 1986. 44 figs. VIII, 169 pp. ISBN 3-540-17073-1

Vol. 132: **Melchers, Fritz; Potter, Michael (Ed.):** Mechanisms in B-Cell Neoplasia. Workshop at the National Cancer Institute, National Institutes of Health, Bethesda, MD, USA, March 24–26, 1986. 1986. 156 figs. XII, 374 pp. ISBN 3-540-17048-0

Vol. 133: **Oldstone, Michael B. (Ed.):** Arenaviruses. Genes, Proteins, and Expression. 1987. 39 figs. VII, 116 pp. ISBN 3-540-17246-7

Vol. 134: **Oldstone, Michael B. (Ed.):** Arenaviruses. Biology and Immunotherapy. 1987. 33 figs. VII, 242 pp. ISBN 3-540-17322-6

Vol. 135: **Paige, Christopher J.; Gisler, Roland H. (Ed.):** Differentiation of B Lymphocytes. 1987. 25 figs. IX, 150 pp. ISBN 3-540-17470-2

Vol. 136: **Hobom, Gerd; Rott, Rudolf (Ed.):** The Molecular Biology of Bacterial Virus Systems. 1988. 20 figs. VII, 90 pp. ISBN 3-540-18513-5

Vol. 137: **Mock, Beverly; Potter, Michael (Ed.):** Genetics of Immunological Diseases. 1988. 88 figs. XI, 335 pp. ISBN 3-540-19253-0

Vol. 138: **Goebel, Werner (Ed.):** Intracellular Bacteria. 1988. 18 figs. IX, 179 pp. ISBN 3-540-50001-4

Vol. 139: **Clarke, Adrienne E.; Wilson, Ian A. (Ed.):** Carbohydrate-Protein Interaction. 1988. 35 figs. IX, 152 pp. ISBN 3-540-19378-2

Vol. 140: **Podack, Eckhard R. (Ed.):** Cytotoxic Effector Mechanisms. 1989. 24 figs. VIII, 126 pp. ISBN 3-540-50057-X

Vol. 141: **Potter, Michael; Melchers, Fritz (Ed.):** Mechanisms in B-Cell Neoplasia 1988. Workshop at the National Cancer Institute, National Institutes of Health, Bethesda, MD, USA, March 23–25, 1988. 1988. 122 figs. XIV, 340 pp. ISBN 3-540-50212-2

Vol. 142: **Schüpbach, Jörg:** Human Retrovirology. Facts and Concepts. 1989. 24 figs. 115 pp. ISBN 3-540-50455-9

Vol. 143: **Haase, Ashley, T.; Oldstone, Michael B. A. (Ed.):** In Situ Hybridization. 1989. 33 figs. XII, 90 pp. ISBN 3-540-50761-2

Vol. 144: **Knippers, Rolf; Levine, A. J. (Ed.):** Transforming Proteins of DNA Tumor Viruses. 1989. 85 figs. XIV, 300 pp. ISBN 3-540-50909-7

Vol. 145: **Oldstone, Michael B. A. (Ed.):** Molecular Mimicry. Cross-Reactivity between Microbes and Host Proteins as a Cause of Autoimmunity. 1989. 28 figs. VII, 141 pp. ISBN 3-540-50929-1

Vol. 146: **Mestecky, Jiri; McGhee, Jerry (Ed.):** New Strategies for Oral Immunization. International Symposium at the University of Alabama at Birmingham and Molecular Engineering Associates, Inc. Birmingham, AL, USA, March 21–22, 1988. 1989. 22 figs. IX, 237 pp. ISBN 3-540-50841-4

Vol. 147: **Vogt, Peter K. (Ed.):** Oncogenes. Selected Reviews. 1989. 8 figs. VII, 172 pp. ISBN 3-540-51050-8

Vol. 148: **Vogt, Peter K. (Ed.):** Oncogenes and Retroviruses. Selected Reviews. 1989. XII, 134 pp. ISBN 3-540-51051-6

Vol. 149: **Shen-Ong, Grace L. C.; Potter, Michael; Copeland, Neal G. (Ed.):** Mechanisms in Myeloid Tumorigenesis. Workshop at the National Cancer Institute, National Institutes of Health, Bethesda, MD, USA, March 22, 1988. 1989. 42 figs. X, 172 pp. ISBN 3-540-50968-2

Vol. 150: **Jann, Klaus; Jann, Barbara (Ed.):** Bacterial Capsules. 1989. 33 figs. XII, 176 pp. ISBN 3-540-51049-4

Vol. 151: **Jann, Klaus; Jann, Barbara (Ed.):** Bacterial Adhesins. 1990. 23 figs. XII, 192 pp. ISBN 3-540-51052-4

Vol. 152: **Bosma, Melvin J.; Phillips, Robert A.; Schuler, Walter (Ed.):** The Scid Mouse. Characterization and Potential Uses. EMBO Workshop held at the Basel Institute for Immunology, Basel, Switzerland, February 20–22, 1989. 1989. 72 figs. XII, 263 pp. ISBN 3-540-51512-7

Vol. 153: **Lambris, John D. (Ed.):** The Third Component of Complement. Chemistry and Biology. 1989. 38 figs. X, 251 pp. ISBN 3-540-51513-5

Vol. 154: **McDougall, James K. (Ed.):** Cytomegaloviruses. 1990. 58 figs. IX, 286 pp. ISBN 3-540-51514-3

Vol. 155: **Kaufmann, Stefan H. E. (Ed.):** T-Cell Paradigms in Parasitic and Bacterial Infections. 1990. 24 figs. IX, 162 pp. ISBN 3-540-51515-1